LOOKING EVERYWHERE
BUT RIGHT HERE

A MEMOIR

LESTER ALAN KALISH

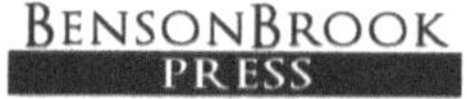

BensonBrook
PRESS

This book is a memoir. The author has attempted to recreate events, locales and conversations from his memories of them and saved correspondence. The opinions expressed within this book are solely his own. The author does not assume and hereby disclaims any liability to any party for any loss, damage, or disruption caused by errors or omissions, whether such errors or omissions result from negligence, accident, or any other cause.

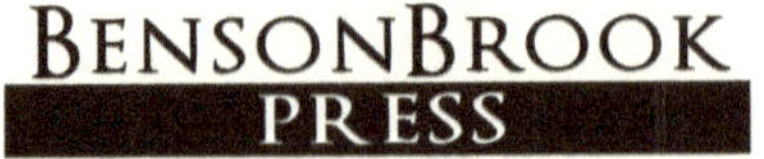

BensonBrook
PRESS

Cape Cod, MA

This memoir is descriptive and insightful. From the beginning, I felt pulled into the story and along for the author's journey of self-discovery. I wanted to keep reading to see what happened next.

-Jennifer Bees, freelance editor

Growing up in Brooklyn, iconic, amusing and moving. A fascinating contrast to the suburban childhood and youth that I experienced.

-Rod McDonald

I found this memoir to be an honest, informative and heartfelt story about one man's journey through the pain, struggles and joy that happens to someone who is navigating the medical and holistic pathways.

- David Young, LMT

I understand how the author lives with the ambiguity of his health status and is open to the possibility that his convictions may change. His expressions of returning to himself, and the image of him and his father in the mirror are powerful.

- *Ronald Wilson*

The poetic novel style that used words to create the experience and atmosphere left me curious and wanting to read more. I appreciate the author's honesty and reflections from a soft and tender heart. His words are encouraging for those in the midst of a difficult season in their life.

- *Beth Thompson*

In my late 40s, I found myself sitting across from my dear Aunt Belle. This frail lady, about to turn 90, never wore makeup, yet her rose-colored cheeks and the radiance of her youth were still visible. An insightful woman, she carried herself with grace and dignity. Everyone was aware that Aunt Belle was nearing the end of her life. As we talked, a comment surprised me.

"I would like to know you better, understand who you really are, what you're really about."

Aunt Belle touched a chord. Knowing exactly what she was saying, I wondered if she could see right through me. I was defensive and so entrenched in my self-illusion that for long periods of time even I believed the masquerade. I made light of her inquiries and chose not to open up to her, even at this late stage of her life.

We sat across from each other in her one-bedroom apartment, Aunt Belle in a chair similar to one my mother sank into for hours at a time, hints of mothballs hovered, reminding me of my grandparents. What I did share with her were my pacifist views and strong sense of justice, along with my building frustration with government and politics. "Aunt Belle, you know I find it easy to question authority." Perhaps this was a generational response to Vietnam and other events of the time. I explained that my environment and demographics college professor said pollution was the biggest threat to our planet. "I was so impressed by this class that I considered a career in environmental studies."

"Why didn't you pursue this?" she asked.

"I don't know," my words rekindling my curiosity.

I thought about mentioning the numerous unexplained phenomena I had witnessed, and how I'd always felt guided, looked after, especially during difficult times. I'm not exactly sure why I didn't talk about this – perhaps Aunt Belle's precarious health caused me to pause. But I knew that I wasn't ready to expose my personal doubts or insecurities. That would take another 20 years to completely reveal.

I have never been comfortable joining and I am not driven to lead, so where does that place me? Well, I march to a different beat and do not want to be defined by anything, especially illness. I love playing in the dirt while planting and landscaping, but I'm not a gardener. I enjoy reading, debating issues, seeking knowledge, but I'm not an intellectual. I was conceived by a Jewish mother and father, but I don't consider myself to be a Jew. I am a mere speck in the universe, mirroring it, constantly changing and reinventing myself. My passion has been a lifelong quest to overcome stereotypes, to learn, to establish and hold dearly to my voice, and to move from intellectualizing to feeling what I know and believe in my soul.

I could not have navigated through the last part of my current journey and stand where I am today without my wife, Mary. She has allowed me to be – to declare like a butterfly emerging from its cocoon that in so many ways, my time has arrived.

Mary's unwavering support as I reacted with utter certainty to the results of a diagnosis eight years ago, one month after we were married, has been a beacon of strength. Bearing witness to what I shared as I continued to learn, absorbing my thoughts and framing my ideas, responding, not judging, walking by my side. "I will always be there for you." These first words Mary spoke as she recited her vows, gave me permission to confirm who I am. Not conforming to traditional wisdom or established mainstream views, or to those in authority who may make decisions without my best interest at heart, as I place a focus on what is dear to me, bringing clarity to my values.

There are many voyages we navigate, connecting to a larger journey, and a number of paths we can take that are influenced by those we meet. Each decision on those roads, driven by free will, dictates the next step. I am convinced that coincidences are small reminders of the miracles awaiting us, if we'd only stop and notice, go within and proceed with an open heart. Can we move through many journeys at the same time? I imagine so, simultaneously learning life's lessons from souls we have agreed to meet, honoring decisions we may have made before we arrived here.

In so many ways, my latest sojourn feels like the most challenging. I have learned that time can erode memories, transforming sensations, feelings and our realities. What felt life-altering or threatening as a young boy would not have the same urgency 40 or 50 years later. A current crisis does not diminish what we felt before; it only changes our perception as we look through a different lens.

This book has helped me connect many dots and view life in different ways, with a new clarity. For this, I am deeply grateful.

If I don't question, I can't learn.
If I don't learn, there are no answers.
If I don't have answers, then I am back to where I began.

1

THE NEIGHBORHOOD

I was 12 years, 2 days and about 3 hours old and — I was staring at Mrs. Bianchi. *All* of Mrs. Bianchi. I may have seen my mother in the shower when I was younger, but this was different.

It was only my second day on the job, that brilliant, sunny, naked-Mrs. Bianchi afternoon. In the five minutes it took me to ride back from Apartment 2R, I rehearsed story after story. You know, the ones we tell our parents that sound so convincing to us and are obviously contrived to them. *The alarm went off! I was stuck in the elevator at the Fontainebleau apartment building for 50 minutes!* This sounded pretty good. Or, *There was a car accident on the corner of Cropsey Avenue and Bay Parkway, blood was everywhere! I helped the couple out of their gray Chevy and waited until the ambulance arrived.* Forget that one – no blood on my jacket or jeans. *When putting away the groceries, I dropped the ketchup bottle. Mrs. Bianchi asked me to clean it up and scrub the kitchen floor.* Not bad, but I'll go with the first one.

With my right hand firmly holding the groceries, I balanced the box on my left knee. My free hand rang the doorbell, which had a strange resemblance to something. I just couldn't put my finger on it. No answer. Minutes later, still no answer but noises approached from inside apartment 2R. As I pushed the smooth, round, red button again, I held firmly while attempting to make it louder. *I can't leave the box outside the door. It might be stolen. I'm supposed to ask to be paid for the order and I want my tip.* However, minutes later, I was resigned to leave, so I placed the box of groceries on the welcome mat and stepped back.

Just as I began to turn, a crack in the door revealed the sounds of a vacuum and a radio blasting a Top 10 song. I moved toward the noise and bent down to pick up the box. As I straightened myself up and looked forward, my lower jaw reached for my toes, my knees turned to rubber, my face flushed, heat overwhelmed my entire body. "Sherry Baby" – The Four Seasons harmonizing in the background mixed with a humming motor, roaring from the gray tubular Electrolux, seemingly moving along like a sleigh. The short cord led to a long narrow pipe, the end sucking dust from hardwood floors – Mrs. Bianchi had no idea.

As my images of Playboy magazines came to life, this slender woman tuned into the music, in her underwear only, no bra, stood there looking past me, oblivious that my world had changed. A surprisingly cold and windy afternoon suddenly warmed up rather quickly. What seemed to take days as this indelible image implanted in my memory forever, ended with a scream of recognition and a slam of the door.

I stood there, my mouth still open for at least 5 minutes hoping to see Mrs. Bianchi to confirm what I witnessed, but also not knowing how to react if I saw her again. A few minutes later I rode back to the store. I was relieved to find my father wasn't there.

That evening my father asked, "Why did it take you so long to get back from the Fontainebleau?"

"You don't want to know. I have homework to do. You can pay me later." I ran to my bedroom. My father never again asked me what happened. Regretfully, I didn't share the story with him as I grew older.

"WELCOME TO BROOKLYN – THE FOURTH LARGEST CITY in the U.S." The simple rectangular white sign with its bold black lettering, as large as car tires, greeted me as I drove across the Verrazano Bridge before I entered the Belt Parkway, as the road turned toward home. I drove my dad's 1962 blue Dodge Dart, pushed buttons on the dashboard to move into another gear while listening to AM radio stations. No cigarette butts or joints in the ashtray – yet.

I was 17, my faded jeans strategically torn or ripped at the knees or thighs, a simple, well-worn T-shirt, perhaps frayed around the neck. Light brown hair beginning to cover both ears, growing longer each day. Looking into the rearview mirror, now clean shaven, I recalled peach fuzz, beginning to appear a few years earlier as I rode my bike or walked the last 2 miles. A paved path, guarded by wrought iron 4-foot fencing, provided protection from the boulders and Atlantic below.

I remember walking in white Converse sneakers, always purchased at Modell's on Flatbush Avenue. Black tar smears from months of stickball games like a badge of honor and worn soles like summer scars comforted me as I moved with pride. Damp days or a northeast wind, hinting that the ocean was nearby, always meant I was home. Moving along, I'd turn left where Bay Parkway begins at the half moon inlet surrounded by rocks, offering up a carnival of amusement rides and fast food at Nellie Bly. Ah, the sweetness of cotton candy, the seasoned smells of fried shrimp and potatoes swimming in oil would reach me as the wind shifted.

I would move along the sidewalk and under the highway, passing a triangular strip of land near the off-ramp, admiring our makeshift diamond – its outfield climbing toward the highway barriers. We'd play baseball here in spring and summer, chasing pitched balls that regularly found their way into the traffic above. With grass-stained knees, as green faded to brown, we'd come back to this hill on shorter, snowy days to sled and watch red skies give way to rising, orange winter moons. Continuing past Cropsey Park, I'd turn right by the Italian deli on Bay 31st Street, my baseball glove in my left hand clutching a Spalding, stickball bat raised above my shoulder in my right hand as I marched in a make-believe army to our block of Bay 32nd Street.

Between five-story apartment buildings on either end of our block in Bensonhurst, rows of single-family brick homes sat separated by narrow concrete driveways leading to the occasional garage. Their stoops and small fenced-in gardens painted the landscape. Two, three or four generations lived under one roof.

Anthony's Soda Fountain stood a block away on the corner of 23rd Avenue, just a few stores from the leather goods establishment. An egg cream made from chocolate syrup, milk and seltzer foaming to a head, or cherry coke were the common requests. We sipped through paper straws while perched on oval red leather stools, turning to look for a friend or to the spot where the new comics were placed that day.

The first time I walked into Bernie's Barber Shop without my dad, four blocks down from the soda fountain, I was intimidated. I looked past the older men, their stubbled faces asking for a shave, searching for anyone I knew and an empty slender steel armed chair, to sit in and wait.

When Bernie called "next" while pointing in my direction, I slid across small piles of recently cut hair and into the barber chair. "A summer cut please," I announced, asking for a crew cut. I sat in a chair fit for a king. Crank after crank lifted me higher and higher until this kind, older man's stale breath of morning coffee and cigarettes made me wonder why everyone liked coming here so much. "My mother gave me this for you." I offered the dollar to Bernie, (75 cents for the haircut and 25 cent tip), who for many years walked past our apartment building on his way to work, his gait and tempo slowly changing as he aged.

We rode our fathers' delivery bike up and down these streets. Since he was older, my cousin Melvin began delivering orders for our fathers' store a year and a half before me. For some unknown reason, once we turned 12 and not a day before, we were deemed responsible enough to place a box of groceries in a metal basket attached to a bicycle and ride blocks and blocks to a house or apartment for 10 cents an order. My first real paying job. It took 11 years and 364 days to celebrate this rite of passage. What a first job!

The bill was a handwritten itemized list with prices, the numbers carried from one column to the next, the total written on the top. "Here's what you do. Take this order to Mrs. Nichols, remove the groceries and bring the box back," my dad instructed. "Give her this bill and collect what she owes if she wants to pay today. You can wait for a tip, then come right back."

I was beaming. I had finally made it.

2

A GRAVESIDE MOMENT

As other relatives roamed the Rebecca family circle plot of land at the New Montefiore Cemetery in Long Island New York, in 1965, my mother and I paused in front of Lillian Kanowski's gravesite. A few months before my 16th birthday, my mother turned 49. As I stood beside her, gazing at my grandmother's grave, listening to my mom read aloud the date Lillian was born and the date she died, an eerie sense came over me, as though I was being drawn into an unexpected reality and, if given a choice, I would resist.

Words in a moment of insight; an unintended lasting memory was formed. "For years I have believed I would die when I turned 56, just like my mother had." These sad words, laced with concern were softly spoken by my mother on an overcast, early June morning. Forty-six years later, what I worked so hard to neatly tuck away in the recesses of my mind and secretly feared, would occur through a slightly different lens.

As Lillian's health was failing, a few months before her 56th birthday, my parents' wedding was hastily planned. All family members including Lillian attended. Shortly after my parents' honeymoon, my grandmother passed on.

My grandfather married his second wife, Fey, a few years later. Isadore emigrated from Russia to the United States in time to escape Hitler's wrath. Other family members were not so fortunate and were never heard from again, their silence leaving a void filled with memories for those whom they knew and stories creating images for those who came later.

A funeral for a family member or to pay respects, placing small stones on the top of gravesites to show that someone had visited and took a moment to remember was always a day's affair. Driving from Brooklyn, the Bronx, Queens, Putnam Valley or Connecticut took hours, no matter what time we left. Tolls to pay, bridges to cross, tunnels to drive through and rush hours to navigate. Planning to be away from life's routine always took a full day.

Following a graveside service for a family member, we would drive back to the immediate family's house to sit shiva on wooden boxes and stools as tears of grief and sadness melted and turned to remembrances and laughter. Food and refreshments to share; cooked chicken, chopped liver, smoked fish, herring in cream sauce, potato salad and coleslaw, challah bread, cookies, sponge cakes. These gatherings supported those who grieved, commemorating those who'd passed.

So many stories of the "old country" were shared during meals or card games. I would watch the adults adeptly shuffle cards, especially my grandmother. She appeared as a card shark. It was a sight to behold as she tossed one card at a time to a precise spot on the table in front each player. Pockets emptied. Piles of pennies appeared like castles of wet sand dropping from our fingers at the shore. For many years I watched and learned how to play poker until finally, I was asked to join my first game. As hard as I tried, I could never beat my grandmother. She always ended up with more pennies than anyone at the table.

I got to know my grandfather as his old age intersected my youth, forming images I carry. Isadore was a big man, large boned, a crop of grey, curly hair that resembled in texture, much to my disdain, my own. My grandfather was the patriarch of the family, also known as the Rebecca Family Circle, which met twice a year in a large hall to elect new officers, address business matters and was a time to play with cousins. As kids, we ran through the halls, drank Kool-Aid, found bags of potato chips and cups of ice cream. This was also a time to visit with aunts.

As though I was peering through a magnifying glass, dark red larger and larger lips moved closer, eyes focused, cheeks round as water balloons, lunged toward me. Outstretched arms and hands encircled my face. Just as an aunt's nose was inches away, she squeezed my cheeks like a fresh loaf of bread. The corners of my lips pressed toward each other, coiled to pucker, "Lester, you're so cute" and then contact! What remained was a slightly smeared, though sometimes perfect painting of my aunt's lips right there on my cheek, my forehead, occasionally my lips, God forbid! Who knows how many kisses were planted on my face by the end of those

Sundays? Yes, my mother, other aunts and older cousins would attempt to wipe it away only to leave it smudged even worse with red, waxy lipstick and lingering perfume; a profound everlasting memory. As I watched my mother push lipstick up through a silver or gold holder, apply it, then place a tissue between her lips to blot, I never understood why anyone would do such a thing. Exuberance was met with reluctance. The long-term effects – overwhelming.

Assured, confident, with a sense of knowing; this is how my mother sounded to me most of the time. Cat-eye glasses, a voracious appetite for reading and crossword puzzles defined her unquestionable intellect. It was natural to believe almost anything she said.

"For years I have believed that I would die when I turn 56, just like my mother had." My father was standing not too far from Lillian's gravesite as my mother uttered those words. It took time for me to internalize her belief, but my mother's haunting words slowly began to reshape my thinking. That single sentence had a profound effect and continued to mold my thoughts; curiosity, watching, waiting. Unintended images crossed my consciousness. Was my mother's destiny approaching? Is she really going to die when she turns 56? This neatly tucked away memory held a dark seed waiting to emerge.

We never talked about this. I was the observer, my mother lived with her anxiety, each of us didn't know how the other's life was affected by belief and a single sentence. I was mostly able to detach from my mother's anxiety, but fear, concern and worry are essentially the same feelings, whether it's your movie or someone else's.

One dark seed gave birth to another. Early spring of 1978,

as my 20s were nearing an end, my father, now 62, took ill. Max had the occasional cold, perhaps the flu. A slight man with a strong body, standing no more than 5 feet 4 inches, he never missed a day of work. Six days a week, waking at 5 a.m. to a shower, shave and a cup of coffee, "Cream and two sugars please." He would walk down four flights of stairs, find two large paper bags filled with rolls, bagels and crullers neatly placed atop a metal cage covering a large hallway heater. He carried them into the grocery store to display in a mesh basket, where they sat for sale, or sandwiches. I learned about the baked goods as a teenager, noticing them when I came home mornings after being out with friends, my father's path and mine never crossing. As I look back, now in my 70th year, fond, long-standing, loving memories could've been formed in that quiet dawn. Regretfully, a missed opportunity.

Shortly after Mom told me that Dad had a melanoma behind his right eye, I found myself sitting beside him as he lay propped up in his bed at Maimonides Hospital in Brooklyn. Conversations followed with Mom and friends. What exactly is a melanoma, what does this mean for Dad's short and long-term health, what are the best treatment options?

Explanations of this disease, scenarios laid out including doing nothing, (which we all agreed wasn't an option), and valuable advice from a practicing ophthalmologist in California, the sister of one of my dearest friends, followed. She confirmed the diagnosis and strongly recommended surgery.

I wasn't part of the many private conversations between my mom and dad, doctors and friends. I imagine how difficult and frightening they may have been. I also know my father's resolve and the faith he placed in the medical profession guided him. Maybe I didn't want to notice the weakness, fear or worry. Perhaps those feelings and emotions were tucked away so all that was visible to me was a man resigned to his fate, accepting and calm. Max never complained. Certainly, in part a product of the times and a trait that everyone who knew him clearly admired and respected.

I am deeply sorry you had to go through this, and I want you to know I love you. I may have said this, but years pass, memories cloud – my journey wasn't yet in sight. I now internalized and began to take ownership of two significant events in my parents' lives; 12 years after my mother's chilling words, my father's discovery that he had cancer stunned me, causing me to pause and reflect.

3

BENSONHURST

rooklyn, New York, 1950s-1960s. The clothesline was pulled slowly toward the living room, into my parents' bedroom, then back to where it hung outside the kitchen window. Latched around aluminum rollers on both ends, with clamps and nails, then joined and tied together. Metal-hinged wooden clothespins had the dual function of keeping baseball cards attached to the spokes of our bikes' wheels and pinning laundry in place. "What happened to all my clothespins?" my mother yelled in my direction. "Must have been the storm last night, they're probably in the alley," I said.

Replacing frayed rope with a newly installed clothesline was an event. Fathers sat precariously on windowsills, their outstretched hands reaching for the line. Three or four stories up, legs dangled above a concrete alley. A window clamped down on their thighs while sitting on the windowsill outside facing in. No net below. My stomach dropped each time I saw my dad tossing ropes or spraying Windex with one hand while he grabbed for a cloth sitting in his lap with the other, then wiped away months of caked grime each spring and fall.

As he twisted and turned, a new rope was dropped from our fire escape to Flo and Bill Sigmond's kitchen window. The line was passed on or tossed through each of the two living room windows, then to the bedroom. Bill would yell over the traffic below, "Throw the line toward the fire escape." Then my dad would scream to me, "Les, send it down to Bill." The clothesline was secure.

I wonder if Flo and Bill's soft-spoken manner and deliberate pace, similar to Flo's father and mother, contributed to their longevity. Flo's parents, Mr. and Mrs. Brown, lived on the fifth floor, walking up and down those stairs every day into their early 90s. As Mr. Brown exhaled, cigar smoke was replaced with a curious look. "Who's better. Mantle or Duke Snyder?" If it wasn't for Mr. Brown, his transistor radio and love of baseball, when the Brooklyn Dodgers moved to Los Angeles in 1957, I probably would have felt orphaned until the Mets stepped onto a baseball diamond for the first time in 1962. Instead of waiting to adopt the Mets, my allegiance turned toward the New York Yankees as the 1957 season came to an end. Thank you Mr. Brown. "I'll take Mantle."

Flo was someone my mom could talk with about my sister, who was born with cerebral palsy that contributed to developmental delays. As Ronda's older brother, the responsibility of looking after my sister began to feel more like a burden. Sometime after I turned 7, it felt like we were growing apart. Yes, some of this was natural, and I did prefer to play with my friends more often at that time, but Ronda's intellectual challenges separated her from most of our peers. Athletically, for the most part, she was able to keep up. She ran fast, had a splendid arm and could throw as far as some boys her age. However, she couldn't grasp many of the rules or strategies involved in our street games, nor the card and board games we would play in the courtyard on hot summer days.

Gradually, as Ronda was not chosen or included with our friends, she began to gravitate toward younger children. At times I was torn, not knowing who to play with, but invariably I stayed with my friends.

I didn't realize it then, but shame and guilt had already begun to surface.

As young children, we stayed close to our apartment building, within the courtyard or directly outside on the street. Our immediate neighborhood was our playground and the many stay-at-home mothers our guardians. Husbands went to work, oftentimes six days a week. Taking a bus, car or train to the city, these mostly blue-collar men brought bread home for their tables. Arriving to soups or sauces, soaking up the rigors of their day in meals their wives prepared, they reconnected in the comforts of their apartments.

Each Monday through Saturday, my father would walk down four flights of stairs, head outside, unlock the cellar and then the gates protecting a door leading to the grocery store he and his brother Abe owned. The store was closed on Sundays. Even though he was one of the few men who didn't travel more than fifty steps to work, my dad wasn't always available to us. A quiet man, he reluctantly offered advice, yet he deeply affected my thinking. His voice was soft, rarely raised in anger.

His facial expressions were occasionally animated but his frequent, radiating happy smile was illuminating.

My dad and I shared hazel eyes and thin yet sturdy body types, with slightly bowed legs. He was always clean-shaven, with long sideburns during the 1960s that later transformed to a cut cropped close to his temples. I didn't know my dad before he lost his hair. "That won't happen to me," I told him emphatically years later, while standing across from the countertop in the grocery store. Little did I suspect my hair loss would mirror his, or that it would not be the only predisposition we would have in common.

Like most children in our lower middle-class Brooklyn neighborhood of Bensonhurst in the 1950s, I began school in a half-day kindergarten. My fondest memory, one of only a few, is crawling under the round arts and crafts table so that I could look up our teacher's poodle skirt. Neil Sedaka's sister was beautiful. Yes, she really was my teacher, however this was not my first crush.

It can indeed take a village, or in this case, an apartment building to raise many families. It didn't matter who was related, if you brought friendships with you or were meeting people for the first time. Heritage, backgrounds, religions all melded with little question or concern. A microcosm of the 1950s in America's cities. Forty-six apartments evenly divided between the A and B sides, all occupied, mostly families with children, a handful of singles, some older parents and their adult children living in separate apartments.

Most of us feared Milty the Super, a tall man with a sneering face and confusing accent. He carried his sour look as he hauled large cans of garbage from the basement to the street for pickup, and as he attended to rusted fire escapes and coal chutes until electric heat was installed. "Stop playing ball in the courtyard!" Curtly spoken words came from the super's open door in the alcove. When Milty was home we took our games to the sidewalks and streets to avoid his wrath.

Izzy was the mayor. No election necessary. An honorary position bestowed upon an elder. Despite being a slight, diminutive man, his presence was felt by everyone who lived in the apartment building at 180 Bay 32nd Street. He just seemed to watch over us. "Iiiiizzy, Iiiiizzy," a strained, high-pitched, aging voice from the third-floor window echoed off the courtyard walls. His wife's call oftentimes was relayed to Izzy, who was attending to his duties street-side. "Iiiizzy, Iiiizzy." Those were the only words spoken as she called her husband for lunch and dinner, and how my image of her was formed. I didn't know her name and can't recall meeting her. She didn't leave their apartment, except when the ambulance arrived one afternoon. We never heard from her again.

SITTING IN BEACH CHAIRS ON THE SIDEWALK IN FRONT OF our apartment building on warm summer evenings, parents and adults shared stories. No air conditioning, the streets became our refuge. A splash of white cement framed the entrance leading to the courtyard. The alcove provided protection from thunderstorms ushering in cooler air, often scattering and thinning the crowd. A ten-foot high ceiling, red brick walls and two doors, one each for a tenant and the super.

Whether outside or under the 20-foot-long shelter, chairs were placed in similar positions each night.

Our entire apartment building packed into cars for the short ride to spend Sundays on the beach. Ten wonderful summers at Coney Island, where bays were distinguished by large boulders jutting out from the shore 100 feet or so into the Atlantic Ocean. Cars unloaded, everyone carried something as we walked under the boardwalk, greeting the cool sand. The line from the shade to sun created by wooden planks was almost as defined as day and night. Not just my feet, but my insides warmed in the summer sun as I emerged onto the open beach.

Sitting on strips of colorful, wide plastic attached to hollow metal frames, beach chairs that sat on concrete the night before now encircled blankets resting on soft white sand. Towels, whiffle balls and bats, all within reach.

Summer Sundays, one bay away from the exclusive Coney Island neighborhood of Seagate, the families of our apartment building gathered at Bay 35. Coolers with Coca-Cola packed in ice, wax paper and aluminum foil surrounded tuna fish and bologna sandwiches on Wonder Bread. Nothing tasted better than that first bite. Peaches, yellow grapes, nectarines, Wise potato chips and thermoses filled with juice. Cigarettes for the parents, plastic jars of soapy bubbles for the kids. The excitement was hard to contain. We ran on the beach, swam, walked on the boardwalk, finding knishes, Italian ices and cotton candy sold at storefronts facing the ocean. Seeing the Good Humor man in his white outfit, heavy coolers packed with dry ice and ice cream strapped over each shoulder, brought joy to us all.

"Just a little further out, let's get closer to that wave coming in," Dad coaxed.

"I'm almost over my head," I yelled.

"Put both feet in my cupped hands, hold on to my shoulders, ready? There ya go!"

My dad lifted and threw me straight up into the air as I raised my hands, placing them together, ready to dive into the ocean. As I wiped water from my stinging eyes, I anticipated this might be the day I would swim on my own. *Am I now ready to go above my head and play with my dad or my friends and swim wherever I want?*

I wondered if the sun would stay out long enough to end this beach day content, tired and aware of the feeling in my throat that said, "This is where I always want to be." The collection of sand, saltwater, and nurturing passed my heart with each breath and radiated throughout my entire body. Inherently, we know what soothes us and the joy of being exactly where we are supposed to be, doing precisely what we are meant to do in that moment. It warmed my soul.

FROM OUR ONE-BEDROOM APARTMENT WINDOW WE could see the rooftop of the Gens' two-story brick home. Their sons were 10 years older than my friends. Consequently, they didn't play with us, nor did Mr. and Mrs. Gen join our parents, but most of the time they didn't seem to mind that we'd adopted their stoop.

Unless we finished supper early enough, affording a choice spot on the Gens' stoop, we were destined to follow a seating hierarchy based mostly on age. Twenty kids could fit on the stoop. The younger you were, seats were found on long, shallow steps leading up to the Gens' front door. The older you were, the higher up you sat. I just couldn't wait for my next birthday. As you stepped onto a 6-inch high painted concrete slab that blended into a garden bed surrounded by black, metal Victorian fencing, your strategy began. The two huge concrete flowerpots – never filled with dirt or flowers – on either side of the stoop appeared as an invitation. They were the two prime places to land, and I imagine I wasn't the only one who dreamt of sitting on one of them. Carved out in red brick above the flowerpot on the right side toward the back, was a concealed long flat area we used as a lounge, always reserved for "tickle torture" – a favorite spot for Harriet and me. Regardless of where we sat, the stoop was a wonderful vantage point to spot the Mr. Softee truck as it turned up our street each night at 7:30.

This stoop had many uses; a free space or the jail for ring-a-levio games, and the best place to play stoopball. "Five, twenty-five, one hundred," we'd call out. Spauldings or Pensy Pinkies, high bouncing pink rubber balls slightly smaller than a tennis ball, rebounded off a step, caught on a hop or on the fly. Whether the ball hit the corner of the step or landed between them dictated your score. For the brave, skilled or risk–takers, hitting the gray and white marble's tiny corner inches from the door and then catching the Spaulding in the air earned you 500 points.

Each time the soft metal screen door was hit, placing marks and dents, a reverberating clink forced everyone to scatter, wondering if Mrs. Gen would come out and yell at us again. If you missed, you ran like hell. "Stop playing!" were the two words we didn't want to hear. Other stoops on our block were used from time to time, but the Gens' was the most convenient and by far the best.

I always wanted to be Mickey Mantle, the Yankees center fielder. He was my idol. Whether playing baseball or stickball, I emulated his stance, hit left and right-handed (because Mickey was a switch hitter) and copied his gimpy strides when I ran.

I could play stickball all day. If there weren't enough kids downstairs yet, I would shoot basketballs at low-lying fire escape rungs, their extended ladders raised as we grew to keep them out of our reach. Or I'd go to another block, waiting to choose up a new game. The tools of our delight were broom handles, black sticky tape on one end and Spaldings, which are harder than Pensy Pinkies but more difficult to control when throwing a curveball.

"Let's hit fungo today." Paul said. You would toss the ball over your head, wait for it to reach the perfect height as it bounced, then swing.

"Can we use a pitcher?" Little Tim yelled. We'd bring someone in from the outfield to pitch. The team up at bat provided the catcher.

A single was any grounder that stayed in the street long enough to pass the infielders. If it hit the wheel of a car or trickled to the sidewalk before then, it was a foul ball. There were always arguments.

"What do you mean it hit the hubcap?" Paul said. It didn't touch anything, get over yourself!"

"I saw it – strike one!" said Andy. A double was a fly ball

hit over the head of the infielders that landed before the Finebergs' home. A triple had to pass the second telephone pole just beyond the Espositos' house on the fly and a home run had to make it to the third telephone pole by the Adlers' house. Any ball caught in the air was an out.

Chalk or soft pastel was used to sketch a roller derby course on the street. Metal roller skates like fitted sandals gripping your feet with skate keys to tighten the hold on your sneakers, gliding along the course or taking to the more challenging, uneven bumpy sidewalks.

Mother May I? A game giving the caller complete control over other children. "Yes, you may take a banana step." "No, you cannot take a giant step." "Yes, you may take two steps backwards."

Hit the nickel, box baseball, slap ball. Spaldings were aimed, tossed, or slapped in an attempt to raise your point total. These ball games were always played to 11 or 21, and you had to win by two.

"Hey Les, gimme that chalk, I'll make a Skelzy board." Melvin had the steadiest hand, so he drew the game on the flattest street surface. Boxed numbers on each corner, a safe zone and dead zone inside a smaller center box. Bottle caps scratched to a silvery smooth surface after dents were hammered out. Then filled with melted, colorful wax crayons and flicked with your thumb, pointer or middle finger making its way around the board. "Wait a minute." As I placed my hand in my back pocket, I felt for the perfect one. I was looking for the 7up bottle cap filled with black wax. I became "the killer" charging to this heavier bottle cap so I could knock everyone out.

My cousin Melvin and I had a distinct advantage. We had first crack at discarded bottle caps that accumulated in the receptacle below the soda machine just inside our fathers' grocery store.

One of my favorite games (and I was really good at it) was flipping baseball cards. It might take a player up to five minutes to complete a turn if he were flipping 75 cards or more.

"I call 74 heads, one tail," Robert announced as he carefully placed a baseball card between his thumb and forefinger, cupped his hands and then let go. When 74 pictures of a player lay face up and one face down, showing only statistics (tails), the next boy would try to match what Robert did with his own cards. If he did so, he kept all the cards, doubling his collection. If not, he surrendered his.

Surrounded by a group of boys awaiting their turn, Robert flipped each card, landing them in what seemed like slow motion on the ground.

"I got next!" someone yelled, claiming the next game.

Cries of "Hey!" "Lookout!" and "Stop!" erupted from our friends; anything to distract Robert and break his concentration.

Paul stepped into the center of the circle after all of Robert's cards lay on the ground. "No problem, I'll match that," he confidently said while flipping his first card.

"Next!"

PAUL, MELVIN AND FAT TIM WERE A GRADE ABOVE Robert, Little Tim and me. They were the leaders of our posse.

It seemed as though it was their responsibility to bring new ideas, schemes and games to our attention.

Fat Tim, "Let's go to the hobby shop and steal something."

Paul, "How about we ride our bikes to the ferry and go to Staten Island? Don't tell your parents!"

Melvin, "Let's play 'Chicken' in that patch of dirt, by the chain link fence across the street."

I hated this game. Two boys stood a few feet apart, facing each other. A Swiss Army knife or steak knife borrowed from the silverware drawer was all we needed.

Melvin explained, "Spread your legs as far apart as you can, I'll do the same. You go first Les. Throw your knife into the dirt between my legs."

"Okay," I said.

"Don't pick up your knife until I move my foot next to it. Good. Now it's my turn."

Melvin's feet were now closer together. As he stood still, Melvin raised his hand and flung the knife between my legs. I turned away, closed my eyes and cringed. Moving my foot toward Melvin's knife, I realized the space between my sneakers was cut in half. Do I throw, continuing the game, taking the chance that some of our toes will not be intact, or end the game? – Chicken.

Between the ages of 10 and 12, my basketball accompanied me as my dad drove his 1956 Chevy from our Brooklyn apartment to the Bronx. Sunday was the day to visit my grandparents and an opportunity to quench my desire to play, run and shoot.

I never knew why my mother didn't learn to drive but suspected it had as much to do with the times (after all, 1950s housewives had other perceived responsibilities) as it did with my father's perception of his wife's ability to safely control a behemoth automobile. Those '56 Chevys were tanks. "Boy would your mother be something on the road," Dad stated on one of our trips. I cannot ever recall an intended sarcasm or hurtful statement from him, but this was close.

Alone, waiting for a game, after a few dribbles, my ball found its way toward the basket. Shot after shot, rebound after rebound, I practiced until someone scooped up my yellow Wilson and hoisted his own shot. It didn't matter that I was picked last or that the ball rarely found me as we transitioned from defense to offense. As my focus and skills improved, I became a "chukker," one who shoots as soon as he gets the ball either for concern that he won't see it again or is extremely confident in his ability. Shots going down, the ball came my way more often.

Sides were chosen, and a full-court game of basketball began. Sounds of sneakers screeching as players pivoted and jumped, landing on the cement, filled the air on these courts in the Bronx. There were few black kids in our neighborhood back home. Though I was the only white kid on the playground directly across the street from my grandparents' high-rise apartment, I was oblivious to race. Whenever I viewed the playground from twelve stories up, through large thinly framed rectangular windows, with its clear view of the Whitestone Bridge and Long Island Sound – all I wanted to do was play.

4

UP ON THE ROOF

At the corner of Benson Avenue and 41st Street, standing in front of the deep red Coca-Cola vending machine, my friend Little Tim and I hid behind our mothers' dresses, their prideful smiles showing no signs of understanding how frightened we were. My mother, Edith, and Little Tim's mother, Dot, urged us along as we reluctantly but carefully looked both ways, peeking back at our mothers, then quickly crossed Benson Avenue and walked the last block together, holding hands for our first day of kindergarten at PS 101.

A week later, we began this 10-block stroll together, without our parents. We'd take the same route for the next six years, missing some days to sickness or when enough snow fell, closing the gates to the large concrete playground and the ominous doors leading to the school's front entrance, its brick dated 1914. Little did we know what would find its way into our lives just a few years from now.

Only inclement weather kept us off the roof of our apartment building. Exciting and peaceful, viewing our world 75 feet above the street below. Drifts of snow would pile against the top railings, like ammunition awaiting the warmth of our gloved hands. We'd throw snowballs as far as we could then watch them land in the vacant lot across the street. Resurfaced hot tar would stick to the sides of our sneakers on summer days. The joy of finding we were the only ones up there – a haven. A chair to sit on, a sun visor to bake under. Looking out over Bay 32nd Street toward Coney Island, the parachute ride was vaguely visible. Tuesday night fireworks, their faint sounds like background thunder, peering through or reaching over trees and apartment buildings, dotted the skies from our vantage point, just one mile away.

The growth spurt that found most of us between age 11 and 16 passed Tim Horowitz by. His younger brother, Andy, touched 5 foot 8 but Tim maybe saw 5 foot 5 when all was said and done. Affectionately known to all his friends in the neighborhood as "Little Tim" because Tim Bochman, a year older and 75 pounds heavier, was conveniently called "Big Tim" or "Fat Tim." An observation and distinction through the eyes of innocent children, the cruelty and insensitivity of those labels appeared to me later in life.

THAT SUMMER OF OUR SEVENTH YEAR, LITTLE TIM AND I left the rooftop, walked down six flights of stairs, into the courtyard and through the alcove, heading for my father's store. Thirty-two years after he and his brother Abe opened the doors, a round stool and the antique National Cash Register would be the two mementos I'd take. Not much inventory remained when my dad turned the key over to Milty. There was no equity – rent was paid for the privilege of running a business – not a penny exchanged hands.

"Please tell your father no beer for my dad," Mrs. Grillo yelled in my direction from their fourth-floor apartment window facing Bay 32nd Street. "A tall one please, Max," Mr. Grillo kindly asked, requesting his signature 16-ounce can of Schaefer beer as he approached the counter. Against Mrs. Grillo's resounding wishes, Max handed it over. My dad had a soft heart and saw no harm in honoring a request from an aging man. "Put it on my tab please," Mr. Grillo would always say in a hoarse, laboring voice.

These cans of beer were ordered for Mr. Grillo only, stowed in coolers with glass doors encased in heavy duty black rubber, hidden behind bottled milk, soda and orange juice. Mrs. Grillo knew how much her dad was drinking because she paid the monthly bill, but this caring charade continued until Mr. Grillo wasn't well enough to walk the streets.

Credit cards became commonplace later. For now, 3 x 5 unlined index cards, alphabetically placed in a green file box by first name only, displayed numbers to the right of dates. Months began a new column. Credit was extended to those who asked for or needed it, perhaps paid back weekly, no interest charge or late fees.

Tiny indents patterned the high tin ceilings. Wooden floors, much like a western saloon minus the sawdust, made their way around a center display that led to the black and white marble countertop. A jar of half-sour pickles, its faded 5 cent sign, stood facing customers.

"Watch this," my dad said while grinning. With ease and grace, he controlled the claw attached to an extended wooden pole to retrieve rolls of toweling and toilet paper, 10 feet up on shelves, softly catching them in his other hand. Canned goods, bottles of ketchup, mustard and relish filled the empty shelves. A stand-alone mesh rack housing Wise potato chips, a 4-foot square tray of candy and gum – attached to a beam seemingly hanging in thin air – enticed children waiting for their mothers. A manual cash register an infrequently used slicing machine added to the cramped counter space.

Two back rooms, one leading to a cold dingy bathroom, the other with an industrial sink (don't drink the water) and space for storage, contained empty boxes set aside for order deliveries.

When he saw me enter the store, in front of Little Tim, the look on my father's face was surprising. Usually happy to see us and never stern, this time we were greeted with a fretted, concerned look. "What were you doing on the roof?"

"Nothing," Tim and I said at the same time.

My dad told us that the leather goods store across Bay 32nd Street on Benson Avenue was a front.

"What's a front?" Tim asked.

"In this case, the leather goods store is not what it appears to be," he explained in hushed tones. "They run numbers in the back room."

"What do you mean they run numbers?" Tim questioned innocently.

"From the roof, did you see a man get out of his car across the street and pick up a bag lying in the grass?"

We nodded.

My dad glanced around the store to make sure he wasn't being overheard. "That bag was filled with pieces of paper with a number written on each one, and a name."

Now I was curious. "What do they do with the numbers?"

My dad explained how people chose a number and paid money to enter into a drawing, so they'd have a chance to win even more money than they'd spent to play the game. This was illegal. He made it exceedingly clear that the man in the car had looked up and spotted us watching him from the roof. "You got lucky this time, but only because you're my son! You don't want to know what could've happened to you," he warned, pointing his finger at both of us. "Don't ever spy on anyone like that again."

We left the store feeling puzzled but fortunate. We had not yet viewed a gangster movie, but we had already been exposed to a dark part of society that we couldn't have previously imagined, and one I would never forget existed. We were introduced to the Mafia when we were 7.

Mid-morning, every day at PS 101, we were given a snack of a wafer-like cookie, and milk. At 11:30 a.m., if you didn't bring food, you joined other children on the lunch line. As Jack handed a $50 bill to the lunch lady in a white uniform for a tray of food, I was curious. The change lady's eyes bulged. "Do you have enough money in the register to make change?" Jack had asked nonchalantly. I'd never seen a $50 bill up close before. *Was it actually real? How long would it take me to save up and cash in my 50-cents-a-week allowance to get one?*

Things started to make sense to me. Jack Marable, always well dressed, an over-the-top charming boy, and James Ricabono, who looked much older and willingly offered a "helping hand," were two of my classmates in elementary school. They never rode public transportation nor walked to school. Each morning, a black Cadillac would pull up in front of PS 101 and let them out. There were no invitations to birthday parties, no playdates. I would only see James and Jack in school.

5

TRANSITIONS

Men were exploring space in small capsules in 1963, President John F. Kennedy delivered his famous speech "Ich bin ein Berliner" at the Berlin Wall, and The Beatles landed, accepting Ed Sullivan's invitation to appear in front of a live audience at Studio 51.

Standing stunned in the halls of PS 128, my eighth-grade social studies teacher Mr. Lipman, was in shock as he told me that President Kennedy had been shot and may die. I didn't know what to feel. When I arrived home that afternoon, I learned that the president of the United States had been assassinated.

The next year brought millions to Flushing Meadows, Queens, seeking the Unisphere at the World's Fair. "A Hard Day's Night" was number one on the pop charts. The U.S. Surgeon General reported that smoking *may* lead to cancer. In 1965, the miniskirt appeared in London, the Voting Rights Act became law giving African Americans the right to vote, and the Rev. Dr. Martin Luther King Jr. led a civil rights march from Selma to Montgomery, Alabama.. With almost 500,000 troops in Vietnam, worldwide demonstrations mirrored those in our own country. Hard to believe, in 1966. the Dow Jones industrial average closed at a mere 785.

The winter of 1967 began with a record-setting blizzard in Chicago that hasn't been matched to date in the windy city. As my senior year in high school came to a close, having traveled only to upstate New York and parts of New England, Chicago seemed as far away as Australia.

Lafayette High School's graduation this spring would take place 25 minutes from home in the Loew's theatre on Flatbush Avenue. My favorite theater, the Benson on 86th Street with a capacity of 1,300 people, wasn't large enough to accommodate 1,375 graduating seniors and their families. On rainy Saturdays or scorching hot summer days, we made our way to the Benson to stay dry or cool off. I ventured out alone one day when I was 8 and sat in this movie house, having spent my 50-cents allowance for a ticket, popcorn, milk duds and M&M's. Ten years later, that's what I would charge students for a ride in my father's car to our college in Staten Island — toll and beer money. My father had approached my seat in the darkened theater. "Where have you been all day?" he asked, whispering in my ear as I sat waiting for the last cartoon to end so that I could watch Dracula for the third time. It would take a few more years to leave the apartment without announcing my intentions or asking permission.

The summer of 1967 was transitional. Mid-afternoon, a warm summer's day, that July before turning 18, college awaited. While hanging around under the L tracks waiting for trains to leave the station, my friends would patiently pause and listen for me to accidentally hit a high note. We'd harmonize to The Beatles, The Beach Boys, The Mamas and The Papas, The Birds and 50s do-wop, our voices blending in perfect harmony – or so I thought. I was drawn to the falsetto tones of Frankie Valli and Barry Gibbs (two of my all-time favorites). On my own, their songs blasting from my transistor radio or phonograph, I joined in, fooling myself for brief moments that I was actually able to carry a tune.

Each and every one of us was a virgin. I knew this because we talked about sex incessantly. After all, we were 17 and we had an agreed upon sign – an acrobatic maneuver –we were all waiting for.

"Is that what I think it is?" yelled Seth Berman. "Kenny Gelb is doing a cartwheel across 86th Street? You know what that means?"

"He's the first to get laid!" Freddie announced to the crowd as we all stood in front of the Florsheim shoe store, amazed but mostly envious.

Boys from the football team sped along in cars paralleling the L tracks, windows rolled down, exposing bare butts, mooning everyone. "Can that be John Elmuccio?" I asked to anyone who would listen.

"How can you tell?" Seth shouted.

We all laughed.

Until then, John's claims to fame besides being captain of the football team were being voted "Joe Lafayette," the best-looking guy in the school, and downing 12 White Castle hamburgers in under two minutes. Known today as sliders; these square burgers on matching buns, from the first fast food hamburger chain were topped with onions, ketchup and yellow mustard. I must admit, they tasted great. I couldn't have foreseen that many years later the shelves in my office would hold books such as The Vegetarian Way and The Vegan Life or that most meals would consist of salads, sautéed vegetables, nuts and grains – no meat, chicken or fish. "You eat so healthy," friends would often say.

We discovered Sicilian pizza, ice cream floats and would challenge friends to eat "The Kitchen Sink," a sundae that would always make you sick. A favorite lunch spot was The Famous, a cafeteria-style restaurant where an assembly line of servers offered up meals selected from rectangular silver trays as patrons called out what they wanted in an orderly fashion, much like high school. Trays of food brought to open tables, shared with strangers and friends.

Chevys, Dodges and Pontiacs dotted this working-class neighborhood. Cars mostly owned by parents were driven by sons and daughters. Parking spaces were at a premium. The shorter the walk to the pizza shop on 86th Street, the more highly regarded you were that night. As weekdays progressed, more and more of our friends would appear until Friday and finally Saturday night arrived, the streets now swelling with crowds from our neighborhood, as well as boys and girls from other high schools.

At the corner Five and Dime store, we would order an egg cream or a Coke while under a dark green faded canopy on Bay Parkway, feet away from the yellow painted stripe that marked the bus stop. A few streets down stood Ebbinger's Bakery, their icing so rich, flavorful and sugary that the cake, always vanilla, was secondary to the experience.

After a night's driving to Canarsie, Sheepshead Bay or Long Island, coming home from a date or party, Jan's is where we met at 1:00 A.M. for a cheeseburger, fries and a cherry coke, comparing how many girls' phone numbers we had or how far we got with our dates. Plans were made for the next day and night, the beach or work, but always back to 86th Street.

When writing to each other in our yearbook (The Legend), or saying goodbye that summer of '67, we didn't quite appreciate how fleeting our friendships were. Four years of our lives; there had been nothing more important than the world we had created inside the walls of Lafayette High School. With a sense of freedom, we reluctantly surfaced to unknown and endless possibilities that last summer. High school friends began to scatter as camp jobs, internships and military inductions took us away from the familiarity and safety of our homes. For most of us, this would be the last time we hung out on 86th Street.

It's funny how it seemed like I disappeared — just like that — with the snap of a finger. *Who am I now?*

6

SEARCHING

My parents' courtship, ignited by a mutual friend of their families, began when my father returned from the war. They kept company for two years. Their relationship, linked by the George Washington Bridge, stretched from the outskirts of New Jersey to the Bronx. World War II morphed into the Cold War and Arab-Israeli conflict. Breaking the sound barrier turned to space explorations and black and white films began to show their colors. As the 1950s approached, a brighter future was envisioned by many.

Twenty years later, there was something eerily familiar about driving my father's Dodge Dart from Bay 32nd Street onto the Belt Parkway, into Queens, across the Whitestone Bridge, entering the Bronx. Those long drives were fueled by excitement and anticipation. Knowing I would be greeted warmly by my girlfriend was as much company as I needed.

A small upstairs apartment in a two-story house, close to 86th Street and the train station, was the first of four places Edith and Max would call home. Home can be a place to remove hats and masks, those we wear as we navigate through our days. Home should be a place to kindle fires of the heart, speak our intentions and share our deepest desires and dreams. It can be a place to raise a family, extend a welcoming hand to a neighbor and watch your children grow. Ideally, it will provide community, shelter as we age, support and compassion. It may also be somewhere we reluctantly call home.

The few stories my parents told me didn't fully explain why they left the apartment in this two-story house. But I can imagine they wanted more space and perhaps more privacy as they planned a family. Just one block away stood their home for the next 35 years, 180 Bay 32nd Street. Apartment 3B on the third floor, the first of two apartments they would rent, had a view of the courtyard from the living room and kitchen, as well as the Gens' tile roof from the bedroom my sister and I shared. The dark courtyard served as a bridge from the street side to the alleyway between our apartment building and a Victorian home on Benson Avenue. A heavy metal door led to the basement with storage space for each apartment, fuse boxes, garbage cans and overhead light bulbs lit by yanking a string.

My father was a man of few words. Raised in Paterson, New Jersey, Max was the oldest of three brothers and one sister. Lou, Abe and my dad were quiet, reserved and somewhat serious men. Abe and Anne were similar in stature. Lou and Max looked alike, they could have been twins. Hints of their Polish heritage defined facial features, a forceful lower lip with an accompanying calm and relaxed expression. They were clean cut, always neatly dressed and moved purposefully. Lou and Max were similar to their dad. I never met my paternal grandmother, but I imagine Anne and Abe, followed her genes more closely. Large-boned, stout, round fuller faces, Anne was more forceful and loved to talk. Abe, the youngest, was happy to sit and listen.

I have always been aware of an unspoken, irrefutable love my dad and I felt for each other. It was easy to get close to him, but there was a more meaningful, deeper connection that I clearly did not understand, yet. When I was a young boy, the difference between Mom and Dad was striking. My father was agreeable, fair, easy to warm up to, but he worked 12-hour days, six days a week. Mom was home more often, so by default she was the disciplinarian. Her confidence and certainty translated to a stern, curt manner.

Mom's weight increased over the years, making it difficult to imagine her as she appears in black and white photos from the 1920s, 30s, and 40s. These photos were neatly tucked into precisely spaced small pieces of triangular paper glued to black, lightweight cardboard in the albums she created. A warm smile introducing large front teeth left everyone wanting to know more. Her short brown hair matched oval-shaped brown eyes, which appeared later in color pictures. No matter the variety of diets, the extra pounds stayed, as did her engaging, friendly smile and curious nature.

"Let's cut a rug, Edie," my father said as he extended his hand. Most people referred to mom as Edith, but my dad affectionately called her Edie. Surprisingly light on her feet, Mom always seemed to be on the dance floor with Dad at bar mitzvahs and weddings. Thanks to the 10-pack of Arthur Murray dance lessons, Dad led, and Mom followed, gliding across the room to everyone's delight.

"What are you doing?" my father asked as I paced around the kitchen of our fourth-floor apartment.

About to turn 18, contemplative, puzzled and confused, I didn't know what to say. "I'm surprised to see you," I finally replied.

"I decided to take a short lunch break," Dad answered matter-of-factly.

It was uncommon for him to leave the store during working hours. At age 10, I'd raced home from Cropsey Park, grasping my middle finger with my right hand. Entering the store, I'd dashed down the aisle holding my broken finger. "My finger, it's killing me. I need to go to the doctor!" I'd screamed in my dad's direction. Playing at the park, a basketball passed to me had ripped out my nail, fracturing my knuckle.

"Wait a minute. I'll call Mom, she'll take you," my Dad had calmly replied, seeing no reason to close the store on my account. "Can I help you, Mrs. Pasquale?"

There was barely enough space for four at our kitchen table, yet it was a place to do homework and hold important conversations while sharing a meal. We sat on red plastic chairs edged with silver tacks. A multi-purpose room, the kitchen was crammed with a large industrial sink, gas stove and oven, washing machine, refrigerator and the chairs. A place for cooking while peering through the kitchen window toward a recently placed basket of clothes. The fire escape also afforded shade from the summer sun.

"I'm trying to find myself," I replied as my father stared at me.

With the world of recreational drugs looming, this catch-phrase often made its way into conversations. We were all looking for something, but I truly felt lost and hadn't a clue what I was searching for. I stood in silence, awkwardly facing my dad, not knowing what to expect.

"Come with me," he said, moving from the narrow foyer adjoining the kitchen toward the living room.

The gray and gold linoleum pathway turned to blue shag carpeting as my dad led me past my mother's high back chair with its ever so slight curve and narrow, stained wood with clawed legs. A cushion to drop into, over time losing its support. Whenever my mother wasn't cooking, working with my sister, or attending to laundry, this chair was like a second home, her refuge. I can't recall ever sitting in it.

A square glass ashtray filled with cigarette butts sat on a small end table with unread books on top of completed cross-word puzzles. A pack of Kents, awaited my mother's addictive clutch. Mom always wore a floral shmata (housedress) and sensible shoes or slippers that exposed painted toes. With a crossword puzzle in her lap, a No. 2 pencil in her left hand, a book between her leg and the chair's arm, she'd be steeped in concentration, unapproachable.

Dad sat on the couch. Except for my mom's chair, their

furniture was upholstered in midnight blue and covered in thick, clear plastic.

I followed my dad past two windows and a television console to the double wooden doors that opened to my parents' bedroom.

"Here son, come over here."

Approaching the free-standing dark stained, full-length mirror, stopping to stare at myself, my father announced, "There you are, you have found yourself!"

Perhaps the most profound words ever spoken by my dad — at least, to this point in my life. But what was I looking for? I knew I was running, but from what? And what was I running toward?

MORE WORDS OF ADVICE

TWO JEWISH BOYS, FRED LEIBOWITZ AND I, WOULD PLAY pool in the basement of Buddy's pool hall with our Italian friend, Donnie Retorto. We'd cruise around, making our way into clubs with false IDs, just hanging out. Best buddies enjoying a slice of our multicultural neighborhood. Fred was 6 feet tall, his fine dark hair always neatly combed, a backdrop exposing large features, brown eyes and cleft chin. Slender, quicker and taller by a few inches, as hard as Donnie tried, he couldn't beat Fred in a game of one-on-one basketball. Although he did beat him many times while playing Horse, showing his creativity.

Two of my closest friends waited in the hallway outside

our apartment. We were 17 years old and this would be our first night beach party at Coney Island. Walking toward the door to let Freddie and Donnie in, I turned toward my dad. A brief pause, a stare.

"Be careful out there," Dad said with hints of a smirk.

We never had "the talk." Sex wasn't a subject we discussed in our house. In those days, you learned about it from older children, magazines, or a girlfriend or boyfriend who was more experienced. I'm not sure if Dad's words were meant to imply that I buy condoms or to treat girls respectfully, or just drive safely, but I chose to believe it was his way of telling me that he had just fulfilled one of his obligations as a parent.

7

THE PHONE RANG ONCE

The birth of an impending snowstorm scattered flakes mixing with sleet, violently pelting car windshields, warning of a mid-winter blizzard. Even when I was a teenager, the excitement surrounding my anticipation of a storm kept me up later than usual.

A phone call so late always prompted a scurry. My parents would rush to pick up the receiver from the beige Trimline phone hanging on the foyer wall before the first ring stopped. It meant only one of two things: someone was in trouble or a family member had died. The policeman on the other end of the line that evening urged my father to come downstairs as he explained the windows of his store had been shattered.

"Edie, I have to go down to the store," my dad shouted over my sister laughing as Bugs Bunny taunted Elmer Fudd on our first color television.

"I'm coming with you Dad," I blurted from my bedroom.

Dad appeared calm yet concerned, as though he was losing

something dear to him. The store was so much of his identity. He was able to financially support our family, which made him proud and it seemed as though everyone knew my dad. The grocery store was a place to stop in and say "Hi."

"How about those Yankees?" Mr. Brown, smiling would say with pride.

"I'm taking a pint of Breyers vanilla ice cream," Mr. and Mrs. Levine would yell while opening the glass doors to the freestanding freezer. Dad would respond, "I'll put it on your tab."

"Long day at work," Bill Sigman would lament whenever he stopped into the store to catch up with Dad after his ride from the city and the three-block walk from the Bay Parkway subway stop.

Bill and Dad enjoyed each other's company. Their common disposition bound their friendship. Many years later, when my own children were 10 and 11, I took them to the old neighborhood. Shortly after we arrived, while standing in the street, as was I painting a picture of our stickball games when I was their age, a car pulled up.

I embraced Harriet as her parents stepped out of the back seat. Appearing as old as Flo's parents, Mr. and Mrs. Brown had seemingly always been, Bill and Flo reminisced about card games, beach days, sitting outside on hot summer nights and Dad's grocery store. With tears in his eyes, Bill told us how fond he was of my dad and how much he missed him.

In the frigid air, disappointed that more sleet than snow continued to fall, signaling the storm had moved closer to us, my visions of mounds of white cleansing the dirt and asphalt vanished. As the storm began to turn to rain, I noticed all the windows had been broken by huge rocks thrown through each one of them. My father's store was no longer protected from the elements.

It's a funny thing. When I think of my friends' parents from the old neighborhood, I remember calling them by their first names. Unless you were an elder or when a so-called friend wasn't really a friend — then their parents were always Mr. and Mrs.

Mr. Bochman, Big Tim's father, sometimes sat next to my dad on hot summer evenings. Mr. and Mrs. Bochman freely joined in conversations, came to my bar mitzvah and were accepted as much as anyone else in our community. Just as the men in our apartment did, Mr. Bochman went to work each weekday. Tall and wide, not unlike his only son, Big Tim, Mr. Bochman was always dressed in well-tailored clothes. He also collected money from my father each month. "Protection" is how my dad described it.

I knew that Bill Sigmund rode the subway to Manhattan to his craft as a dental technician, as did my uncle, perhaps catching the same train to sell shoes in New York City. Little Tim's father sold fruit. Paul's dad was a butcher. I didn't know where Mr. Bochman went each day, or if he was somehow connected to the leather goods store across the street, but as I grew older, I suspected.

What I did learn is that my father had either forgotten to pay "protection" that month or was just fed up having to share the little he made with a strong-armed enforcer, representing the antithesis of hard work and clean living that my dad aspired to. The look on Dad's face, sadness and resignation, as he stood in front of those broken windows, glass scattered about his feet, fueled my anger. My dad was being intimidated by a bully's father. What a wonderful role model.

Feeling protective and invincible, this 17-year-old urged my dad to tell me everything. Wisdom and a desire to protect me prohibited him from sharing all he knew about the Mafia in Bensonhurst. Enraged and determined, a sense of responsibility emerged. Somehow, I was going to look after my dad.

Is a man able to be discreet out of fear for his family's safety and the prosperity of his business? Given a choice, are you a man if you carry this within to keep the peace? Are you more of a man if you expose the truth? I imagine these were some of my father's thoughts and concerns, perhaps framed differently. I can still feel his anger and disappointment.

A month later, after the store's windows were replaced and winter's grip began to loosen, I was walking home from Lafayette High School, approaching our apartment building, when I noticed two police cars parked on Benson Avenue. Our school's claim to fame was the senior production, "Sing" which gave us an opportunity to participate in the chorus with the sole purpose of meeting girls, and a former student who pitched for the Brooklyn and Los Angeles Dodgers, Sandy Koufax.

I spotted my dad sitting on his wooden stool looking pale, frightened and visibly shaken.

"When the man pointed a gun at my head," my father told the police, "asking for all my money, forcing me to the floor, cutting the phone lines, cleaning every bill from the cash register, and told me not to move, I did exactly what he said."

Seeing him in this shocking state so soon after his store windows were broken fueled my desire to protect my dad even more. I desperately wanted to look out for him. And I wondered if there was a connection to what happened that cold winter evening.

As a junior in high school, this spring I was studying for the PSATs. My father and I had agreed if I was at home and he grew suspicious of someone in the store, he would ring twice and hang up.

I was slow to get up as the first ring turned to silence — another one. I reached for the phone, a long pause, then recognized that this wasn't a call I had missed. *Oh shit! This must be our signal.* I hung up. Running down the stairs hastily thinking about what to do, not knowing what I would find, fresh images of the holdup intensified my anticipation. Stopping short of the narrow doors, I slowly entered the store, looking down both aisles.

As I made my way to the counter and joined my father, I spotted a stocky man with dark hair walking toward us. An elderly woman was busy examining canned fruit. I couldn't read the look on my father's face – was it surprise, concern, confusion?

Knowing the long thin knives to slice plastic from salami, along with larger knives to cut bread, were hidden from view under the counter, I carefully felt for the largest knife I could find. Driven by adrenaline, unable to think clearly, concern for my father's safety and perhaps a bit of redemption, I pulled the knife out as the dark-haired man approached.

The elderly lady screamed, adding color to frowned concentration and lines of age. The man looked stunned.

"What are you doing?" my father yelled.

"I thought – the phone – it rang twice. I rushed down. I thought you were being held up again."

Recognizing the absurdity of this while attempting to calm the stunned woman, my father introduced me to his friend, Frank. Relieved and a few laughs later, we agreed to abandon this phone plan.

8

THINGS HAPPEN FOR A REASON, OR DO THEY?

There was something following Little Tim, perhaps an unpaid debt, karma. Mishaps found my friend too often.

"Faster, faster, put your hands in front of you! Make sure you push off the silver square on top," yelled Melvin. Three feet off the johnny pump, with a running start, picking up steam as you approached the fire hydrant, reaching in front of you, bracing your hands on the top bolt, hoisting yourself two, three, four squares of concrete forward, flying through the air. "Oh no!" we all cringed. As often happened, Tim hesitated, stumbled and landed squarely where it hurts boys the most.

A few years later, I was introduced to the jockstrap and the cup, before my first Little League baseball game. Where were they when Little Tim needed them?

Firecrackers were strategically placed in what began as dog food, after making its way through the digestive system and then deposited on the streets. No pooper-scoopers in the 1950s. If you were chosen to light the firecrackers, your exit had to be swift unless you stumbled and landed on the ground, as Tim had, just inches away from the exploding remains. What a mess!

It got worse. "Let's go into the empty lot," Paul encouraged us to cross the street and begin our ascent.

Climbing the chain link fence to retrieve Spaldings or search for lost treasures was always exciting. The idea was to make your way 6 feet to the top, carefully placing your hands between the twisted wires, either jumping over and down to the other side or carefully avoiding the sharp edges as you slowly climbed down.

"I can't look!" Paul cried as he turned his head, closing his eyes.

Little Tim had lost his hold and his lower lip was caught on the protruding top edge of the fence. He was barely hanging on with one hand, his right foot wedged into a small diamond-shaped hole. From where we stood, it looked like he was hanging by his lip. It took 20 stitches to stop the bleeding and hold Little Tim's lip together, leaving a reminder that was visible throughout our childhood.

JUNE 1957

My mother and I were greeted by a large, older man wearing a white patch over one eye underneath his glasses. Strips of partially torn surgical tape attempted to cover any signs of a bulging, ailing eye and kept tears from streaming down his cheek. He was imposing and a bit scary at first. But, Dr. Sadowski, our new family doctor, listened to me.

Our conversations had little to do with health after this initial visit and he was interested in most anything I wanted to talk about. He was the first person who really listened – it was nurturing.

Every other week I walked five blocks to his office and took a seat in the waiting room. No matter how many patients were there, he always had time to talk. "Hop on the examination table and hold on to the painless bar," he said with kindness. This strip of metal covered with white tape kept the pain from the allergy shot away. As I handed over five dollars and watched him toss it into his bottom desk drawer, we'd continue our conversation in his cramped office.

Dr. Sadowski also made house calls to our apartment when we were too sick to go to his office. I can still smell the rubbing alcohol as he opened his leather physician's bag and feel the burn and subsequent ache in my butt from a shot of penicillin. No painless bar in his bag.

He was a true country doctor living in Brooklyn.

"Please God, somebody do something! Where's the ambulance?" pleaded Dot, Little Tim's mother. "This isn't happening, someone help my son, please!"

As a child, summer sickness at best is miserable, at worst intolerable. More often than not, colds or allergies would take their toll, keeping me inside. From where I stood in our apartment on the third floor, viewing the Gens' rooftop from my parents' bedroom, the sky was clear blue. Squinting through watery eyes at the bright sun, feeling the closeness in our house (no air conditioning), it felt like another hot, steamy, summer day and I was confined to the apartment – once again.

As I moved to the living room, I tried to make sense of the faint cries of confusion, terror and fear filling the air from the street below. The aftermath of this dreadful accident wafted toward our open window, its concave, black metal guard facing the courtyard and alcove leading outside. Even though I was spared being witness to what I have pieced together from stories and my imagination, I can still hear Dot's wrenching screams as she stood in sheer terror, begging for the car that hit and ran over her son to be removed.

The feats of strength and heroism that followed, perhaps from my cousin Melvin or his dad Abe, or maybe my father, Bill Sigmund or Mr. Bochman. The scurrying to get blankets and towels to quell the bleeding, to keep Little Tim warm and to cry into. The inordinate amount of time it must have taken for the ambulance to arrive. The concerned look on everyone's face; friends, parents and others who'd heard the cries and ran toward them.

Time heals in many ways. Months after the accident, toward the end of that summer, I was able to see Little Tim only once during his hospital stay. Twenty-four-hour vigilance, ice baths to keep his temperature down, antibiotics to prevent infections, and surgeries put Little Tim back together. We were 8 years old. Little Tim and I were best friends. I felt scared and awkward upon entering the room with its view of the Belt Parkway at Coney Island Hospital. Little Tim was sitting up in his bed, Dot beside him in a chair. His parents ushered me into his temporary home for the last two months. As healing and hope replaced my apprehension, our parents smiled while they talked with Ronda. Little Tim and I grinned.

"Are you okay?" I asked.

Tim replied with a shrug, "Yeah?"

His voice seemed different, weakened, sad. But as we talked, fear melted, and I knew he was going to make it.

Nine years later, Little Tim turns onto Bay 32nd Street in a used Alfa-Romeo. "Hop in. Let's go for a ride in my new car." As I sat next to Tim, I could tell he recently learned to drive a standard. Just a few feet from the site of his accident, while moving into second gear, Tim's left foot dances from the clutch to the brake as a young boy darts into the street on his bike. As fenders clashed, for a brief moment I existed in an alternative reality.

The boy was okay, the bike was dented – I could only imagine what went through Tim's mind.

Selling fruits and vegetables near Coney Island, Hy put in long hours to provide for his wife and their two sons, Little Tim and Andy. If Hy had a day off, it was during the week. He never took part in the occasional Sunday outings or our beach days.

Dot, slender, agreeable, her high-pitched voice freely joining in most conversations, sat outside in the shade of our apartment building on Bay 32nd Street on those hot summer days, joining other mothers, watching their young children as they played. As if the director of a movie ordered a scene change, mothers all rose at once. Their chairs, knitting bags, containers of fruit and drinks all moved with them into the afternoon shade across the street by the empty lot as the sun crossed the sky. Everyone sat on concrete squares 5 feet or so away from the chain-link fence.

Sharing an August birthday 20 days apart, Little Tim and I came into the world in 1949. Andy was born five years later. A happy time as we celebrated his brother's birth. Our friends running and playing, Little Tim's cousins, aunt and uncle rejoicing, all gathering in their one-bedroom apartment a flight down from ours. Like so many families in our apartment building, siblings shared a bedroom until a brother or sister became too old to sleep in the same room. If their parents could afford $25 more a month for a two-bedroom apartment, the younger sibling slept on the Castro Convertible in the living room. Thank God I was the oldest.

"Steel on bone" should have been the motto, not "So easy to open, and very comfortable, even a child can do it." I wonder if Bernadette Castro ever slept on one? A U.S. Senator later in life, as a young girl of 4, her iconic television commercial ran more than 40,000 times.

The few times I slept on a Castro, I was awakened by a piercing jolt while I searched for a softer place to sleep. The only thing worse than sleeping on the pullout couch with its inflexible, cold steel frame and thin mattress, was attempting to get up from the couch's clear plastic on a hot day without making a sound, like peeling tape from paper, and with as few red marks on the backs of my thighs as possible. Plastic was everywhere in those days; on chairs, couches and sofas, making it impossible to stay dry. Couch and chair preserved, dignity and comfort sacrificed.

1962

A short time after Dot passed on, and a few years after Hy died, both from heart conditions, the air was heavy with grief and loss. I found myself walking from the same kitchen I played in eight years before, to the living room with Andy's unmade bed. To the small white hexagon tiles in the bathroom directly across from Little Tim's bedroom. As we moved through the apartment, I offered to help clean, organize and find empty shelves for canned goods, boxes of cereal, bags of chips and spaghetti, all sitting out on the kitchen table, bought from my fathers' store on extended credit.

Little Tim was 13, Andy was 8 and somehow, with the help of their aunt and uncle and the parents and friends in our apartment building, Little Tim took on the inconceivable task of raising his younger brother while attempting to walk with his grief and sadness, trying to make sense of his tragic life. *If things do happen for a reason, please tell me why.*

Not always knowing what to say or how to express my regrets and compassion, many days of walking to school in silence followed. With a fondness in my heart, over time Little Tim and I found our separate ways, graduating high school, moving on to college, finding our places in the world.

"You were and have been the best friend I had my whole life." After losing touch for 40 years, in an email that grew out of a Facebook birthday posting, Little Tim wrote those words at the end of a letter recounting his life since we last saw each other at his wedding in Texas, when we were 28. What seemed so important to us at the time – our friendship – had faded even more quickly than the memories of a little boy facing life or death. Much too soon.

9

INSTINCTS, LOVING WITH ALL MY HEART

Our relationship, mother and firstborn, was anything but easy. From all accounts, the first 15 months were blissful. I was happy, except for the occasional colic and being surrounded by cigarette smoke resulting from two packs of Kents a day, my mother's only vice, a gray smog that always seemed to hover within our tiny apartment. Feeding on demand, bodily functions addressed, regular baths, naps, being read to, making faces, rolling around and learning to walk. How great was this?

When my sister showed up, on December 26, 1950, everything changed, and my parents' celebration became my irritation. Developmental delays contributing to social challenges and a low IQ separated my sister from her peers. Her dark, hazel eyes offered a standing invitation and a warm trusting gaze made it easy for anyone to approach her, including animals. She loved them all, particularly dogs. Growing into an attractive teenager, reaching 5-foot 6, Ronda easily related to children years younger than herself, joining in games we had played when we were 7 or 8.

The apparent innocence of the early 1950s matched my joyful existence. These times were fresh with new discoveries. Television; Howdy Doody; huge baby carriages with silver moldings, axles and shock absorbers; Perry Como; Elvis; the Slinky; Mr. Potato Head; and corner grocery stores.

The average family had one TV, one car and 1.6 children (really?). In our neighborhood, almost every family had two children, including my own. The occasional only child showed up, but no one cared.

I loved Rene Wurtzel. I would like to say there was something about the way she walked, the way she looked at me when we played, even the way her name sounded, "REE-nee." But at the age of 4, I had no idea what attracted me to her. Unknown forces drove me to walk up to the fifth floor where she lived. I found her in the hallway and told her I had something to show her. I don't remember if she screamed, bolted or just gazed in curiosity. Perhaps she simply stared at my penis peeking through my zipper because she was an only child - no brothers to educate her.

Is that why she chose Mark to date in high school and eventually marry? I doubt it. Even if I knew at 4 my actions would create a lost opportunity, I believe I would have acted as I had. It was just the thing to do at that time. I wanted to share an important discovery, something I was proud of, with the girl I loved. If this wasn't loving with all my heart, then I don't know what is!

Once again, I gave my heart away. This time I was 11, about to turn 12. The fullness and richness of love comes later, when memory, desire, gratification, dreams and a deeper understanding of who we are drives us to find a life partner. At 11 years of age it's much simpler. When the purity of uncomplicated love finds you for the first time, the only option is to try it again. The hard part is finding the right person and knowing when to take the risk.

As innocence, instincts and guidance led me to that fateful night during the summer of 1961, I had big plans. The one vacation week a year my parents took, getting away from the concrete sidewalks, steamy streets and the grocery store brought us to the Young's Gap Hotel in the Catskill Mountains. When we arrived, I met a girl the same age as me. Linda and I were inseparable.

Memories of these vacations are filled with new friends, swimming, fishing and the smells that came from fenced-in cows standing roadside swatting flies with their tails while grazing on fresh cut grass. Rolling hills, mountains and lakes bellowing with frogs and crickets. The rumbling of thunder toward the end of the day, so far removed from where we were that it might take 30 minutes or so to make its way to us as we counted the seconds between lightning strikes and claps of thunder. There were new games to learn and share, tractors plowing, corn to pick while walking near a field, raspberry and strawberry patches. From the kitchen's backdoor the cook offered freshly baked cookies, sandwiches for a day's picnic and bait for your fishing pole along with a welcoming smile.

The days ended too soon. There was always more to do, and I had the energy and desire to run, to propel myself through the air as high as possible on splintered wooden swings or choose up a game of softball. As evening approached, showers washed away what was left of the day. Fresh clothes and wanting appetites made their way to shared dinner tables. Oftentimes, roaming performers entertained.

Linda and I agreed to meet down by the lake one night while our parents were attending a show. We kept our secret rendezvous from everyone. Back in my room after dinner to change, the excitement and anticipation rose. I didn't know why I was feeling this or exactly what it was, and I didn't care. I was riding a wave that was taking me places I had a sense of once before. No plan, no desired outcome, a faded earlier memory guided me. This also felt new and fresh and something beyond myself moved me along. It was a wonderful, instinctive ride and no amount of deodorant could prevent my underarms from staining my white button-down, long-sleeved shirt. Fortunately, my white sweater acted as a buffer. Matching white pants and sneakers completed the look.

My stomach rattled, emitting strange noises as I walked on the damp grass from our cottage to the lake. My wet palms mimicked the grass. My mind raced so quickly I couldn't remember anything. Destiny awaited me. Drawn to take off my sweater, I discovered by now that my armpits and shirt were one sweaty mess, however, this didn't prevent me from placing my sweater on the grass behind Linda who was standing facing the lake, waiting for me.

While we sat listening to crickets and bullfrogs, a chill came over me. As hot as it can get in the Catskill Mountains during the day, temperatures can drop rapidly when the sun sets. I found myself moving closer, being led by something beyond me. I felt compelled to place my arm on Linda's shoulder. The heavy cool moist air vanished, my heart raced as my hand pulled us closer. In a flash I knew what I had to do.

Time suspended, innocence was about to be transformed, my lips were ready. It was quick, it wasn't pretty, and I got lipstick! Sheer disgust and repulsion revisited as my transition to manhood paused. I had to leave. I don't remember if I said goodbye or if I walked Linda back to her cottage.

Embarrassing letters followed, sent to our home address, were delivered to the grocery store. Humiliating because the letters were received by my father, Uncle Abe or cousin Melvin – and they did take every opportunity to bring them to my attention. Letters with perfume and SWAK written in plain sight. Yes, kisses of lipstick! Instead of using a tissue, Linda used an envelope addressed to me. Lipstick! To this day, I will not kiss my wife if she is wearing lipstick or even Chapstick on the coldest, driest day of the year. Thank you, my well-intentioned aunts.

***

Known as Rusty before we met in high school, my red-headed friend Steve and I enjoyed spending time together. From ages 17 to 20, we took turns driving our fathers' cars, spending weekends away at our girlfriends' houses. Hanging out on 86th Street or playing golf (I was always Arnie – Arnold Palmer – Steve was always Jack – Jack Nicklaus), shooting pool or basketballs, we engaged in friendly competition. Steve was the captain of the track team. Even though I would become an avid runner in my late 20s, we never ran together, but our lives would parallel at times, separate, then intersect again, always aware of the other's presence. Steve has been a source of new experiences and inspiration. Carefree best friends talking, listening to music, deciding who might stay over and how each of us would make our way back to Brooklyn.

WITH MY SIGHTS ON HOW I WOULD BENEFIT, CONFIDENT and cocky, this 18-year-old schemed to take Sandy away for a long weekend by ourselves. We had been dating for two years. My persuasive abilities were on display as I approached her parents and convincingly made a case for the two of us to go away. Lying about spending three days with my parents in the Catskill Mountains, I was somewhat surprised when Sandy's mom and dad agreed. Calling a hotel, I registered as husband and wife. Blinded by my own desires, I actually believed we would pull this off. As we approached the shared dining table I realized we didn't have wedding rings. "Let's keep our left hands under the table while we eat," I said to Sandy. It was an awkward meal – everyone had to know.

THE TENZERS' MIDDLE DAUGHTER HAD SIMILAR challenges to my sister. Their younger daughter, Valerie, and I began seeing each other after I turned 19. I could see how kind Valerie was with her sister, yet I was reluctant to spend time with Ronda. Valerie was in high school, my first year of college in Staten Island was about to begin – we were two and a half years apart. Being emotionally immature, I felt more comfortable dating younger women. It gave me a false sense of being in control. Feeling inadequate and insecure at times around most women my own age, relationships typically ended after a few dates. Seeing Valerie for two years kept me artificially close to what I was running from.

A year after we met, I convinced Valerie's parents to let her accompany me to Haiti while I studied the country's culture, in particular voodoo. This independent study provided the credits I needed to graduate college with a degree in psychology and sociology. I was driven by passion and my persuasive abilities stemming from childhood. I felt invincible.

With both Sandy and Valerie, I wanted to steer the relationship. I used my charm but was still confused and believed our feelings were reciprocal. I grew out of my late teens into my 20s seeking selfish pleasure. In a strange and curiously unhealthy fashion, I was close to my girlfriends in ways that I couldn't be with my sister and transferred my reluctant affection from Ronda to them.

The cool hippie with well-groomed hair concealed my insecurities during the mid and late 1960s. Rallies and demonstrations provided opportunities to express our displeasure with government. We stood for causes we were passionate about. However, by now, identifying with any group didn't interest me as self-doubts drove my ambivalence. I have never felt comfortable outwardly associating with a large group, even though our views or values may have meshed. Difficult to identify when driven by a false image.

A few years removed from college, with three or four jobs behind me, attempting to save money, I continued to distance myself from my family. Working in sales, doing what I was meant to do at that time in my life - what came naturally, I believed I was ready for a mature, nurturing relationship.

Could this be true love? What I had thought was real love brought me closer to true love in my mid-20s. I met Janice at the Concord Hotel in the Catskills. Her mother had died when she was a young girl. Raised by her dad and older brother, Janice graduated with a degree in education and taught at a school for the deaf. Empathy and familiar circumstances brought us closer. We shared road trips, new friends, light hearts, an apartment, and visions of our future together.

It was so easy to be with Janice but, saying "I love you" began to feel like a habit. Out of obligation or promise, these spoken words gradually lost their intended meaning. The intensity diminished, their binding strength weakened, they become mere words to reflect upon, concluding and questioning whether and how deeply I loved. I wasn't able or ready to make a commitment and to love someone authentically yet. At 27, after four years, our relationship ended.

10

CONFUSION

My neuroses and anxieties stemming from my insecurities would be fairly developed by the time my own children would come into the world. Many nights I would check on them a number of times to make sure they were breathing – until they were 8! When my wife was pregnant, I strongly urged her to change her diet and lifestyle to give us the best chance to have a healthy child. This gave me a false sense of control. I didn't want to relive, as a parent, what it was like growing up with my sister. In my private moments, I wondered if the universe again would nudge me to try to learn to love in the face of adversity. During these times, I prayed.

Parents hover over their firstborn child. They can't wait to hold her, watching her sleep and dream. They spend time observing their firstborn, looking for milestones – first smiles, words and steps. And they learn so much about themselves as they instinctively respond to their children's needs.

But the firstborn is different. The smells and cooing are so fresh and new. You just have to spend as much time with your baby as you can – not that subsequent children don't bring much joy. However, the addiction can change as abruptly as it began when a child's sibling arrives a year or so after she was born. The focus begins to shift to the newborn and suddenly the first born is no longer the center of the universe. Efforts are made to create a balance, but circumstances can make it nearly impossible to sustain. Newborns demand so much time and attention, it's only natural for the firstborn child to feel left out, saddened or wanting, lonely or afraid.

Time freely spent and sought after abruptly turned to a longing. Will I be left alone again? When will this end? Of course, my parents had good intentions, but my mom and dad faced unexpected challenges shortly after Ronda was born.

I would like to say that I have a memory of how and when I began to feel abandoned, but all the years of therapy fell short of taking me that far back. In fact, it's impossible to remember much before age 5. It is certainly feasible that the time before kindergarten was so traumatic that I buried that tape. But what I believe is that I began to learn how to get my way at all costs, demanding and independent as my personality unfolded.

ONE MORNING IN 1956

Alone in my bedroom, crying out so God can hear is profound; asking for something, then waiting and feeling disappointment is heartbreaking. Can you feel this at the age of 7? "Please God, help Ronda, make her like me. I know you can hear me!" Perceptions can change, time will erode memories and certainty may turn to doubt. But I do remember looking skyward, eyes tightly closed, head down after searching through clouds, imagining I could see God. It probably was only one prayer and at that time was mostly for my sister. I knew Ronda was different, something wasn't right, and I didn't know what else to do.

I don't recall conversations my parents may have had with me that centered around Ronda's challenges, and how they viewed my role. But it seemed like Mom and Dad were insisting I care for and look after my sister. As a young boy, even if I was able to completely understand, I didn't want this responsibility. I just wanted to play with my friends.

It was all on me to live up to my potential and difficult to express how that made me feel, so I rebelled against subtle signals of higher expectations. With firstborn hopes and promises, and a second child with special needs, assumptions that I would succeed heightened. I acted out at times, afraid to ask for help, struggled in elementary school, and in some ways identified with my sister, not knowing if something was also wrong with me. As time moved on, I felt more distant from my parents, particularly my mother. Wanting to be seen and recognized for who I was, but reluctant to expose anything hinting that a fragile, confused, wounded child lurked inside, my perplexing identity continued to take shape.

Even though my parents did love me, I felt compelled to disguise my confusion and need for more love with a tough guy façade. Moving into middle school, sharing some classes with older struggling students, raging hormones added to my bewilderment. I believed I was fooling everyone. But Philip Carlo, the most feared boy in school, saw right through my mask and fortunately decided to look out for me. Finishing Philip's wooden penguin in shop class helped and afforded me some protection.

Challenged to an after-school fight, frightened of what would happen to me, I shoved my mask in my backpack and raced out of school as soon as the final bell rang, taking a different route home just to make sure I wouldn't be seen. The next day, walking through the halls side-by-side with Philip, no one dared come near me. This may not have been the best choice of disguises for a frightened, sensitive boy, but it's one I felt drawn to construct.

An actual fight between Vinny and Philip took place a week later, across the street from the middle school. Students gathered near a gated garden, the combatants inside. It didn't take long for the blood, hatred and violence to melt my mask and send me home even more confused, not knowing how this 11 ½-year-old boy should present himself.

A few years earlier, while being harassed by Big Tim (who picked on this skinny kid whenever he had a chance – like father like son), I found myself running. Being chased, realizing Big Tim couldn't catch up, zigzagging across streets, I gathered speed and reached out for a metal pole with its "NO PARKING TUESDAY AND THURSDAY" rectangular sign hanging like a flag. Grabbing onto it, Big Tim approaching, I turned in his direction. We clashed head-on. The force knocked me over as Big Tim fell to the ground.

To my surprise, landing on top of my pursuer and childhood tormentor, much like Ralphie did to Scott Farkus in the

1983 movie "A Christmas Story," I began to hit then punch Big Tim. Revenge in my hands, tears of joy quickly turned to remorse. I was not a fighter and we were now even in my view. With mixed feelings, I left the scene crying. I can still hear the kids in the neighborhood laughing. Were they laughing at a cowardice bully being put in his place? Or, was everyone making fun of me?

In my mid-20s, while attending my cousin's wedding, walking into the banquet hall with my girlfriend's arm in mine, I noticed Bill and Flo, my cousins Melvin and Robert, many friends from the old neighborhood, and Big Tim. Thrilled and excited to introduce Sharon, we walked toward everyone. With an enthusiastic hello my arms flung around Big Tim, having long come to terms with our childhood relationship. He quickly moved out of my grasp with a look of disdain. Big Tim frowned, showing his true colors. Once a schmuck, always a schmuck.

Four years later, now 31, a cold New Year's Eve, on the Upper West Side in Manhattan, I left a party with my date. Exiting the elevator, moving into the lobby, brushing the arm of a man walking by us, spontaneous, angered looks turned to punches. My troubled, perhaps drunk attacker taking out whatever rage lurked inside him, wrestled me to the ground. Reacting in defense, I held my own. Realizing there was no battle to be won, my opponent left. I stood by the elevator stunned and shaking, surprised by my actions. Not really knowing what had just happened, people from our party responded to the noise, racing down the stairs to my aid. Back inside the apartment, supported by my new friends, I cried. I did so for a long while, many tears and years later, reinforcing what I always knew. I'm not a fighter, I'm a lover – and still confused. Masks may change, but the lost child still hides behind them.

———

MY MOM WAS NOT OFTEN AVAILABLE – BOTH emotionally and physically. Much of her absence centered around learning how to best address my sister's needs and becoming a trailblazer for children with disabilities. There were numerous conversations with parents comparing progress, sharing newly discovered therapies and attending Board of Education meetings to encourage the creation of special classes. Saturday night bingo games in a long bygone movie theater in Sheepshead Bay were just one of the many fundraisers established to support their work. Talking and sharing, always with an eye on what the future would hold.

I learned about Willowbrook in Staten Island, New York, viewed by many as the standard of care for the mentally challenged at that time. A disturbing story by a young reporter, Geraldo Rivera, was broadcast in 1972 on the Channel 7 news. Images of children and adults wearing similar white gowns, roaming stark empty hallways searching for a place to sit, finding corners of sterile rooms, staring or shaking with virtually no one to attend to their needs, were horrifying and disturbing. This was not a place my parents were going to send Ronda!

My mother wanted to include Ronda in everything as well as to find other families whose children had similar challenges. She worked tirelessly to teach my sister to read, calculate and write, spending hours and hours with cue cards, props, penmanship exercises and important life skills. Along with the help of other parents and professionals, my mother would find her way. Born and raised in the Bronx, my mother Edith Kanowski, had always wanted to be a teacher. She never finished her degree, but her desire was fulfilled, skills utilized, and passions practiced with her second child.

My sister's education would be remedial at best and work opportunities scarce. Helping to support organizations like the American Association for Retarted Citizens and others, my parents began to accept that Ronda would most likely spend her weekdays reinforcing basic skills, sorting items, enjoying arts and crafts projects, and socializing in a sheltered workshop.

"I hate you! I hate you! Leave me alone!" Ronda yelled in my mother's direction.

"You're not doing it right, turn the pencil around in your fingers, like this," my mother, relatively removed, suggested.

"I don't love you. I want you to go. Leave me alone!" Ronda screamed.

"Do it your way. I don't care anymore. What's the use?" Mom yelled back.

My father stood, visibly upset, torn between whom to calm first. I wanted to run. Sometimes I tried to explain to Ronda why Mom was trying to help her, often to no avail.

More arguments ensued, my mother's rage blending with frustration and guilt, eventually yielding. My mother steadfastly sustained her efforts long after the state was required to provide education. Congress enacted Public Law 94 -142, The Education For All Handicapped Children Act, in 1975, three years after legislation was introduced and six years after Ronda last set foot in a school building.

Ronda in her early teens to late 20s, Mom in her early 40s to late 50s, it was a difficult time when a variety of medications were introduced to calm my sister. For a long while I believed this to be unnecessary. But I later realized they were vital to manage inappropriate behaviors. My sister continued to live with our parents into her mid-30s. The time together in their home classroom diminished when Mom began working part-time, and eventually full-time as a bookkeeper. What would my sister do as my parents aged?

Most children climb the school ladder to their senior year, happy to leave home for college, returning for a visit during semester breaks and holidays. Eventually, the time comes to move out and raise their own families. But parents with special needs children would have to consider a group home or find another family member willing and able to provide care. Many hurdles my sister would face were unknown and could only be addressed as they occurred; biological milestones, illness, parental sickness as well as learning to accept separation when alternative living arrangements had to be made. As a community rose out of concern and a common quest for answers, the needs of my sister and her friends with similar challenges were matched by love from everyone in their extended family.

If these nurturing groundbreakers were able to glance at

the future, they would have been astounded and pleased to discover the many advances in place for developmentally delayed and intellectually challenged children and adults. They would know that their efforts prompted others to continue focusing on the needs of this population.

Edith, at nineteen, after two years at Hunter College in the Bronx, a country still reeling from the Great Depression, with war in sight, had to leave college to work and abandon her pursuit of a teaching degree. It took her away from her dream and closer to the reality and struggles of the times. She had no idea that her most valued student would later be her daughter. As war approached, Edith would find her two brothers enlisting and a changing world with new priorities.

World War II was the end of Max's education as well. After graduating high school, while working at the Big Bear Food Market in his hometown of Paterson, New Jersey, a precursor to what would be my father's vocation, he enlisted in the army. While serving two years as a private first class in the South Pacific, he unknowingly awaited the birth of the nuclear age. Max arrived back in the states four months after the attacks on Hiroshima and Nagasaki. I have pondered the effects of nuclear fallout on his health and believe the exposure to a contaminated far-reaching environment may have expedited the growth of cancer in his body, as well as so many others – too soon.

11

FINDING THE QUIET WITHIN

Is it possible to come to a decision when external noise and internal chatter churn? Cars and buses carried people, trucks delivered goods, pedestrians moved about, fire engines, an occasional ambulance, the L tracks three blocks away. Life in Brooklyn was noisy – to say the least. I'm not sure when I first noticed the city buzz, suppressing how the sounds felt, placing them within, attempting to block out distractions.

Childhood to 23, living three or four stories above the street below, renting an 8th floor apartment in Kew Gardens, Queens, a room off Main Street in Yorktown Heights. In my 30's, the first home I owned was on an elevated hillside near enough to Route 84, the sounds of cars speeding down the highway in either direction was a constant source of irritation. Years later, a home in East Greenwich, Rhode Island, a mostly quiet neighborhood, but directly in an airport landing pattern. Planes on descent seemingly brushing the tops of telephone poles – advertising their airlines, the roar of jet engines vibrating as they slowed down to land. Now, on Main Street in Orleans, Massachusetts, cars race by, police sirens lead to tickets, summer workers talk with friends while riding their bikes after our dreams have arrived; lawnmowers, construction, concerts and baseball around the corner in the park.

Times with my parents and sister in the Catskill Mountains, vacations to secluded beaches, retreats in the Berkshires. I always find quiet welcoming. Stillness, peaceful times to reflect, listen, move inward. The contrast is obvious.

As a young boy, I was easily influenced. Music, breaking waves settling on shore, conversations not meant for my ears. The ethereal sounds of a cantor's voice moving me Saturday mornings. I may have stepped into a synagogue three or four times after my bar mitzvah. From age 9 to 13, I went to Hebrew school late weekday afternoons. Occasionally I attended Saturday services and joined my father in prayer during the high holy days of Rosh Hashanah and Yom Kippur. Carrying plastic bags filled with bread, each fall we'd walk past Nellie Bly to the guard rail and toss stale pieces into the ocean atoning for our sins of the past year. Happy New Year.

I discovered transcendental meditation in my mid-30s, a reminder of how I have attempted to escape from external and internal jabber. The quiet within felt like a gift. Synthetic means, mostly marijuana in the 60's and 70's, beer or wine later, helped bypass the prattle. If I had it to do over again, I would take more time to be still, recognize my inner voice, trust my intuition, and breathe.

My mom's fervent words that day at the New Montefiore

Cemetery, my dad's first serious illness. Having to decide what to do about the draft in early 1970.

———

DECEMBER 1969

The draft lottery was televised – 365 balls, numbers that were coded to match birthdates haphazardly tossed inside a tumbler like popcorn in its machine. When August 24 dropped into the slot and was subsequently announced, I knew a decision had to be made. The 36th ball to fall meant I had to report for a physical. Pending the results, do I join the Army, the reserves or go to Canada and avoid Vietnam? Time to stay still, reflect. As my morals evolved, beliefs raised questions and doubts surfaced.

Shortly after my cousin Melvin joined the Army Reserve, he convinced me to go to a recruiting meeting. A cavernous space, the armory in Sheepshead Bay was cold, threatening and void of compassion. As soon as I walked through the huge doors leading to evenly spaced, dated, grey metal desks manned by soldiers in uniform, I had a burning desire to flee. Run from the stories, newspaper articles and my imagination. Run to my innocence, not wanting to surrender it too soon. Run to the safety of parents, friends, the comfort of our apartment. Run from bureaucracy. Run from the government who ignored a majority view, fueling the industries and lobbyists who had the politicians' ears.

Run to what I believe, to my strong conviction that there wasn't ever a single reason that made any sense to wage war. I always felt there is no rational explanation for suffering, hatred, killing, tragically upending families, destroying cities, towns and neighborhoods.

I've never viewed the battlefield as a place for heroism. True heroes are watching out for their young children at home, caring for their families and aging parents. Dedicating their time in communities, cities and countries around the world. Humanity is what they stand for.

When will we learn to love in the face of differences, to put them aside in the name of peace and allow our children to thrive in a nurturing world? Heroes step forward out of need, react instinctively or perhaps feel they have no choice. We call attention to their sacrifices on the battlefields of manufactured wars, and without them, most assuredly, more men and women would be lost. But, why do we portray heroes in the context of war?

Heroes can be defined by choosing to stand for a greater good and challenging governments that continue to fight anywhere a cause can be made to infuse resources that can be better used to fight poverty and disease. They can argue that these means should not be used to create more weapons to point across boundaries, ideologies, religious beliefs and so-called principles. Courage is refusing to fight for any reason except in defense of decency, humanity and for those we love. Even then, I want to believe there is a better way!

Words of reason and acceptance, building foundations to appreciate contrary views and celebrating differences – that is what heroes stand for. Searching for what unites us – not pursuing an enemy. Someone has to say no, refusing to take up arms. Many have, since that first battle on our planet hundreds of thousands of years ago began, sending out waves of disharmony for all in the universe to hear. I know this may appear naïve and difficult to conceive, given the state of the world as we know it, but just for a moment reflect on what it would be like if we all decided to stay at home with our families? What would happen if no one showed up to fight? If each one of us was a true hero? What would our world look like? I venture to say, closer to heaven on earth than finding yourself facing life or death on a battlefield – much too soon.

I wasn't about to go to a foreign country in the name of democracy and peace and attempt to kill a so-called enemy I didn't recognize. Were my convictions strong enough to follow in the footsteps of a famous African American, refusing induction, deciding to surrender 3½ years of his storied boxing career? The country was divided. Not everyone viewed Muhammad Ali as a hero, standing for what he believed in.

Questions surrounding my manhood, courage and pride in country surfaced. *If this was WWII, would I volunteer or serve if I was drafted? How grateful am I that I live in a democracy but how much faith do I place in my government? If I have the right to freedom of speech, by extension do my words give me the right to abide by my thoughts and values?*

As we sat around our kitchen table, my father urged me to consider moving to Canada if things didn't go as I hoped it would at the draft board.

Dear Mom and Dad, Bill and Betty,

What am I doing here? Why did you let me come? I regret not having a full life to appreciate what I now know I feel, wanting to act out of love. I'm lying here in a ditch by myself. Most of the bleeding is over. I don't have much time left but I want you to know I am beyond the terror. I'm not confused anymore. I know I'm going to die. I am sorry I didn't have a chance to raise a family or be an uncle.

I regret that I enlisted and came here to fight. I don't know who I wounded or killed. I don't know how many families are homeless and how many children are missing because of my actions.

The heat and humidity are fading. I feel cold. Grief and heartbreak surround me. Like morphine running through me, I am calm now. I know I will be left behind, and my memories will fade. Darkness seems to be turning to light, and I hope I can return with a chance to make amends. The next time my actions will stem from love and will ripple like the rings in a pond, touched by a stone tossed from the soft hands of a child.

Maybe next time I can really make a difference! I love you for bringing me into the world. I'm sorry for any pain I have caused.

John

A LIFE FADED AWAY AS QUICKLY AS THEIR NEWBORN SON'S first wide-eyed smile turned from innocence to curiosity, to confidence then independence.

Wailing and sobbing met me as I knocked on the 16th floor door of this high-rise apartment building in the Bronx. When my girlfriend Sandy opened the door, tears streaming down her face, cries poured from her parents' bedroom. The knock on her door earlier this day brought the news that Sandy's brother John, Bill and Betty's son, had been killed in action. Tens of thousands of times, letters handed over by officers in uniform. "Your son has been killed in action serving and honoring your country." "Your son is missing in action while serving and honoring our country." The flames of hope and dreams detonated by a mine or bullet. It could have been me.

The Vietnam War didn't have much time left in 1970. Protests and chants of peace took place around the country a mere 25 years removed from World War II, and even less time since the Korean conflict. Too many boys had to act like men. Not enough of our young were buying into a divided country's request to serve.

I found myself following lines of boys stripped down to their white Fruit of the Loom underwear, except for the occasional pair of red or pink panties, moving from station to station. "Keep your head straight, move your eyes left to right, stick out your tongue." "Drop your drawers, bend over, turn your head and cough." Commands to follow orders, all in an effort to see who was fit to serve.

Straight, fine, long brown hair to his waist, Jesse built hot rods three blocks from our apartment building. During the physical he screamed for everyone to hear, "I am the son of God!" Drinking a flask of red liquid, he proclaimed, "I am swallowing the blood of Jesus Christ." Jesse didn't serve, nor did any number of boys with the creativity or courage to stand up to the establishment.

Allergies and asthma, words like food sensitivities and seasonal disorders stood out in the letter I handed to an army officer from Dr. Sadowski. I saw parts of Canada when I visited, later in life. I also chose to subdue feelings around courage and conviction for a while.

When I was 8, five years before the Cuban missile crisis, at the height of the Cold War, our teachers scheduled a drill. We hid under wooden desks near a window in elementary school. In 1957, the concern for our safety radiated from our teachers. Fear, fright and confusion weaving in and out of our lives.

Is this really happening? As I turned on the radio, sitting in my Honda Civic after a 9 a.m. appointment at the Oxford Middle School in Connecticut. I was tuned to the Imus in the Morning show. I first thought this was just one of his bits. Imus was talking with Warner Wolf, a sports reporter who was painting a horrifying picture of planes crashing into burning buildings, people jumping out of windows. It didn't take long to realize this wasn't a script. It was an actual attack on our country. I rushed home, called my wife, and waited on the front steps outside our red clapboard, colonial home in New Milford for the school bus to arrive with our sons.

While sitting shaded from the afternoon sun, shocked, confused and worried, realizing that September 11 will be a day not soon forgotten, I became enraged. In some ways, I was reliving through my children what it must have felt like for my dad, his brothers and sisters and their parents when Pearl Harbor was attacked. These thoughts were so daunting and powerful, the feelings so raw and frightening. Has anything really changed?

A RUDE AWAKENING, A MAJOR SHIFT

1*976.* What would it be like without my father? Shortly after learning my dad had cancer, I visualized for the first time what it would be like if my father died. The stark reminder that I, too, will die changed my life. Based on old habits and taste, until this time, I didn't care much about what I ate – a piece of meat, french fries, bread, beer, an occasional glass of wine. Fried eggs, toast and hash browns were my choices for breakfast. Lunch consisted of deli meats, mayoladen tuna fish or fried foods.

Everything changed when I internalized that the one man on the planet whose unquestionable love I shared, was not invincible. I didn't feel this deep connection with my mother or sister, but that would change as age and illness found their way into our relationships. It had been much easier to love my dad. Now, I was startled. Death became all too real. Just like that, within a flash, the first 27 years of my life didn't count. Or so it appeared. Who am I now? I began to see things differently and my priorities shifted. My self-centered, pleasure-driven focus was replaced by a desire to learn about nutrition, exercise, conditioning and prevention. (Of course, I was still in my 20s and some old habits would take more time to break.)

A new journey began one hazy, Friday August afternoon at the Bronxville High School track. Ego and pride prompted me to run at full speed. I had played basketball, football, stickball and baseball in the streets of Bensonhurst and the parks near the bay, always competing, never tiring. Once an athlete, always ready to throw, catch, shoot and run. Yet, I barely made it halfway around the track that day.

I removed my gray sweat-stained shirt, wiping away perspiration and what was left on my face from throwing up. White Converse sneakers with little support, a red stripe above the sole, shin-high white socks and no water bottle. Twenty-seven and horribly out of shape, I left the dirt track and walked home. Disappointed, embarrassed, but still determined, the warm moist air hovering overhead accompanied me as I trudged through the winding hills back to my apartment in Tuckahoe, New York. But it wouldn't be the last time I would lace up my sneakers.

As my mother moved past 56, I began to identify more with my father and his timeline. My mother's words that day at the cemetery now had an accompanying mantra, "I don't want to follow in my father's footsteps." The seeds of my doubts fed a slowly mounting neurosis. I was determined to do everything in my power to prevent disease from finding me in my early 60s as it had my dad. I felt driven to break old habits and live a healthy life. In the fall of my 27th year, I began a serious quest to let go of concerns of my own demise. I was determined not to have to consider similar decisions my dad would face during the next 10 years of his life.

MY TRANSITIONAL 30S, RELATIVELY STABLE 40S AND stormy 50s were in front of me. A series of experiences and relationships would help reframe my focus. Trading three-piece suits, matching shoes, $30 haircuts and a sales career for newly purchased camping equipment, I ventured across the country. With my 30th birthday on the horizon, I had six days to drive to California and drop off the car I had been hired to transport. I made my way north to Niagara Falls, west to the Dakotas and south to Colorado, through Las Vegas into California. My journey began with just enough money and food for the week – and a vial of cocaine.

As I was pulled over, cars speeding by on Highway 89 near Lake Powell in Utah, I wondered if I had time to hide the evidence.

"Do you know how fast you were going?"

The police officer then asked me if I would like to sit in his air-conditioned car while he wrote my ticket. I had been moving through his state at a modest pace, 90 miles an hour or so, and it was scorching hot. No air conditioning in my car.

"Sure, thank you." Sleight of hand accompanied my response as I tucked the little glass cylinder into the seat crevice, sliding a loose towel on top of it.

I never paid that ticket.

A week later, viewing parts of my life through a rearview mirror, I made my way home.

Upon my return, with a 10-day growth of facial hair, not realizing over the next 25 years age would be marked by gray streaks in my beard as much as my thinning hair, I stepped into a new life. Having enough money in the bank for a while (or so I thought), no debt and no direction, the excitement of my newfound freedom gradually eroded. Relishing not having to get up at the same time every day turned to staying up late and awakening as morning touched noon. No foresight or planning, the future was as far away as – well, the future. I barely looked beyond my nose.

Little discipline to define me, searching through books such as "What Color is Your Parachute?", attempting to rediscover my passion, and find a direction, savings melted as quickly as winter abated. I drove my car into the ground, turning to my bicycle until flat tires forced me to walk. I was spiraling. The time came to move from my apartment in Tuckahoe to Yorktown Heights, eventually settling in a small cottage in Putnam Valley, New York.

Looking for what I lacked, believing I needed to fill a void, it seemed as though wherever I found myself – a business meeting, bar, supermarket or gas station – I desired to connect with a woman. To talk, stroke my ego and hopefully develop a relationship.

Shortly after turning 31, I was working at Nor-West, a

recreational facility, planning and implementing programs for developmentally challenged adults. Fifteen hundred miles away from my sister, who was living with my parents in Florida, I was attempting to unleash guilt. While attending a conference that addressed the challenges of the physically impaired, I was intrigued by one of the speakers. From afar, sitting at the back of this banquet hall, I was smitten with a bright, wholesome, articulate woman.

Making my way toward the stage as Joy's presentation ended, I suddenly stopped. Seeing her slowly walking from behind the podium, grasping two crutches, then moving to an awaiting wheelchair gave me pause. Do I continue holding onto my hopes, abandon them completely, or praise Joy for her courage and moving speech?

I didn't think my ambivalence was evident as I asked, "Will you join me?"

We sat at a table and talked. Looking into her spiritual blue eyes, desiring a connection, I felt enticed to move closer.

Visiting her parents' home, meeting our friends for dinner, carrying Joy into my town's community pool for a swim – we built a relationship based on admiration, fondness and caring. But also, an underlying hidden truth lurked – that on a fundamental level I was functioning as I always have - confused.

A beautiful woman who shared deep thoughts, expressed her emotions, desires and passions had strong feelings for me. I couldn't access those same feelings. But being superficially close to Joy made me feel whole. I was still searching through others for what I lacked – my ability to be close to my sister. Joy and I were acting out this human drama at the expense of her open heart.

Realizing I couldn't continue this charade a few months after we met, I found myself in a strange bed one night in an empty room alone – distraught, engulfed in shame, falling into depression. I didn't know it could get so dark. I had to change, face my own reality, embrace it, attempt to move past this. Four months after we'd met, I regretfully said goodbye.

STEPPING IN AND OUT OF RELATIONSHIPS DESTINED TO end, still feeling lost at times, I began noticing my neighbors Bill and Maggie's love of gardening, John and Nancy's joy of Muppeteering and other people's passionate energies surrounding me in a small community of 12 cottages in Putnam Valley. I spent time with Maggie, learning ways to sculpt the soil to produce food for my table, and worked at a summer camp directing plays for children with disabilities. I taught cooking classes and adapted equipment for physically challenged adults at a nursing home. During this year I began to unlock my creativity that lead me to a conclusion.

While working at the Knolls Nursing home in Valhalla, New York, Keith, a soft-spoken, gentle man who later became my roommate, introduced me to Mary Altieri. Ten years younger than me, Mary was home for summer break from college and worked as a nurse. We began dating. As the days shortened – calling Mary back to school – my infatuation heightened and prevented me from clearly seeing our time was coming to an end. What I felt, however, stirred my creative juices even more, guiding me to my next career.

13

APPRECIATING STABILITY, COUNTERING UNCERTAINTY

I was confident it would be easy working with children who had similar challenges to my sister – it felt like a natural fit. So, I enrolled in graduate school the summer of 1981 and began working toward a degree in special education. What was I thinking? My soul laid dormant and cried at the same time. Hired as a full-time substitute teacher at BOCES, in Yorktown Heights, New York, I took an extensive course load, completing my program in one year. I began my first teaching position in the fall of 1982.

I envisioned a fulfilling life, especially when Janet and I met a few months before my final semester. Stemming from love, pride and a desire to let my father know the family name will carry on, I asked Janet to marry me. With my 36th birthday in front of me as we planned our wedding, we were aware of cautionary signs that would play a role in the years to come. Janet is levelheaded with an even temperament. She provided a steady income throughout our marriage, but I could not be counted on to do the same. My dad's declining health prompted us to be married in Florida. Although my father would be with us for more than two years after we were pronounced husband and wife, the resemblances to my parents' wedding were striking. Once again, my mother played an important role in the planning.

Recently out of graduate school, my first teaching position a year old, life had much to offer and Janet and I were poised for an exciting ride. Our first son came into the world a year and a half later. Seven pounds six ounces, thick black hair touching his temples, a round face (mostly cheeks) and brown eyes. After 36 hours of labor, Janet's huge sigh accompanied Bryan's appearance 10 days after he was due. Fourteen months later, blue-eyed, blonde haired chubby Evan, weighing in at 10 pounds 6 ounces, his face even larger than Bryan's, decided it was time to join us ahead of schedule. We barely made it out of the hospital elevator as Evan viewed the world for the first time.

We spent five years in our first house, a small Cape with an unfinished second floor. As our family grew, the house seemed to shrink. The summer before Bryan entered kindergarten, we moved to a larger colonial with more room, and subsequently more debt, just as my teaching career began to show signs of uncertainty.

Familiarity can be a stepping stone to a place you want to be, but it shouldn't be the most important consideration to stay. Moving to a different school district with new responsibilities didn't change what my soul was trying to tell me, and my heart inherently knew. While there was much reward and personal growth, as well as benefits to those students in my classes, my passion and desire dwindled. Instead of being with my sister, I ran. By working with developmentally delayed and learning challenged adults and children, I attempted to deal with my guilt.

I wasn't looking forward to teaching in what would be my last year and had not taken the time during the summer to prepare to work with a severely handicapped child while piloting a newly created inclusion program. The first day of the new school year was to be a challenge. It turned into a disaster. After 15 years in special education and my 40s nearing an end, a telling moment began to unfold as I drove to school.

Sharp cutting pains resonating from my lower back almost brought me to tears. Entering the principal's office, nauseous, pale and sweating, I waited for a ride to the hospital. Discovering my kidneys were being attacked by calcified stones, after several hours the doctor sent me home.

Two subsequent attacks, each time passing out in the back of an ambulance in horrific pain, kept me home that fall more often than the days I spent at school. Having much time to reflect, I found the school district questioned my credibility and dedication. The universe was getting my attention and the signs became clear. Shortly after I passed the stone, it was time for my teaching career to end. I left teaching in June of 1998.

ANOTHER ENDING

Eighteen years is a long time. It didn't take long after Janet and I met for me to realize I was rewinding a familiar tape.

Attractive, petite, reserved, not one to readily share her feelings, subtle reminders surfaced, in particular the distance I felt from my sister. I couldn't offer Janet everything she would hope for in a marriage. Still, we were compatible in many ways. So much so, doubts faded, and we embarked on a life together, creating meaningful memories and bringing two wonderful children into the world.

Time with siblings, vacations in Maine with parents and grandparents, dinners out, biking, sharing the excitement of a new house. Horseshoe games in our backyard, children growing up together, and neighbors becoming better friends.

I believe it's inherent to seek happiness, to feel complete and whole. Eighteen years is also a long time to stay together, particularly when the responsibility of raising children becomes the main focus and financial burdens take precedent over time alone. We allowed the wrong reasons to surface and the right ones to fade.

As the distance between us grew, I was unaware of what occupied my wife's thoughts and continued to search for what comforted me, knowing our marriage would soon end.

When marriage goes beyond its time, it's easy to forget who you are. I suppose if my dad were standing next to me, he would have asked me to step in front of that mirror. Chasing fading dreams, knowing they won't come true while attempting to rekindle old flames, distractions shifted our focus. We weren't able to find solid ground as the world Janet and I had created slowly crumbled. We were still joined, more by fear of the unknown, security in what we possessed, remorse for the truth behind our appearances and worry for our sons, than love, honor and respect for each other.

A few years into my educational consulting business and one year and a few months removed from meeting our collaborative attorneys, saying "I do" to the judge when she asked if we accept everything in our divorce agreement, Janet and I were officially not married. Eighteen years after we'd said our vows, made our promises and celebrated our wedding in front of family and friends in Delray Beach, Florida, we parted.

Furniture divided, personal items stored away for another time, the house felt like a shell. On the road for 35 to 40 hours a week, and just as much office time, I worked to keep the house that Bryan and Evan had lived in since they were 5 and 3½ years old, allowing them to finish high school with friends they grew up with and attempted to build something new from something aging. I found time for an occasional retreat, yoga classes, running, of course more wine and encounter groups in Charlemont, Massachusetts.

CHARLEMONT, 1992

Having an out-of-body experience can change your life, literally. The life you know stops existing and where you find yourself isn't quite clear. It's like being between two worlds. "How do I integrate back into my life?" I asked my good friend Steve – a practicing therapist – who along with Nancy, was co-facilitating a group of 12 people during this weekend retreat. He suggested, "It's impossible to expect what you have taken away from an encounter weekend to sustain you indefinitely."

This small group formed a society bound by curiosity and attempts to listen and talk with others, allowing vulnerabilities to surface, exposing anything we felt. It can be extremely intimidating. It was like live theater without a script.

A simple concept, somewhat bizarre. A dozen people sat on old, worn but comfortable couches in the great room of a dated farmhouse on 20 acres of land in western Massachusetts. All watching and waiting to be asked to join another person. Eventually, someone would break the silence. Two people would move to the center of the room, like a stage, facing one another, gazing into each other's eyes, reacting to what they felt. The intensity of these encounters reached each person in the room.

"Can I place my hand on your heart?" Nancy asked while we sat on the floor.

"Yes," I responded.

Within minutes, my eyes closed, deep breathing becoming shallow, I left this place. I didn't know where I went or for how long I was gone. I don't remember anything but a hand gently landing on my shoulder. Sometime later, reentering my body, I slowly opened my eyes and noticed Nancy's inquisitive look.

"Where did you go?" she asked.

"I don't know," I said.

As I attempted to remember, I asked who had placed their hand on my shoulder.

"No one," Nancy said, as others confirmed.

"It was the most loving, supportive touch. It felt like the

hand of God," I said, with tears in my eyes, as I attempted to make sense of this.

That weekend, as well as others, with the support of like-minded souls, I was able to experiment with this new way of flying.

Later that evening, Nancy asked me not to move into a trance-like state and leave the group during a session. I didn't do this purposely but did learn, by deep breathing with intentions of "astral traveling" I can do just that.

14

A PROMISE AND A LOSS

If we were told and believed with absolute certainty that we would die in 10 years, what would we do with our lives?

Ten years – that's how much time my dad had from the day he first learned he had cancer to the day he would pass. He was told a melanoma behind his eye would alter his life, leaving him at age 62 with no option but to see the world through his left eye only. My dad agreed to surgery. What did he know, or suspect would happen? How did he feel as time passed? My dad generally didn't share much, and I imagine he may have retreated further into himself.

Smoking two packs of cigarettes a day, little exercise or concern for nutrition, dairy night every Friday, meat dishes, fried foods. These are just some lifestyle choices that could have brought my mother's fears of dying at 56 to fruition. When I discovered my father had cancer, letting go of what I perceived as his invincibility, as well as my own, I realized I didn't want to be subject to the same fate – learning to live with a cancer diagnosis. I began to see 62 as a potentially frightful time in my life. It seemed so long from now, more than 20 years from where I stood. When something is so far in the future, it's easier to let go and live your life. *Don't worry about it, tuck it away* I repeated to myself whenever random thoughts reminded me of my dad's plight.

I was about to get a glimpse into how my dad felt and was shocked to hear what he was about to share. Three years from his first surgery my dad faced another health challenge.

"This is a curse," he said softly while slipping into a fog, the anesthesia beginning to take him away.

"What do you mean?" I asked as he lay in a hospital bed, minutes from being taken to surgery to eradicate prostate cancer.

"Your sister," my dad whispered. As his voice faded, the anesthesia rendered him unresponsive. I yearned to ask more.

I witnessed my parents as they nurtured and supported Ronda, as well as the tumultuous times and confrontations that always seemed to take place between my sister and mother. I was stunned to hear my dad's words. I had no idea he held onto underlying regrets and disappointment.

Relatively good health followed, allowing my dad to enjoy some of his time in Delray Beach at the Kings Point Condo, where new friends gathered in the clubhouse for dinner and a show. Art classes, poker nights, mahjong, golf and swimming were activities my parents enjoyed. However, my dad still missed the old neighborhood. Not the cold, but everything else. "It's okay down here, it's better than the cold, damp winters in Brooklyn, but I just can't get used to the sirens," my dad shared during one of my visits. "I often see ambulances moving elderly people from our condominium to a hospital. It seems to be going on all day and into the night," he sighed.

———

MID-DECEMBER 1986, FOUR MONTHS BEFORE MY DAD Passed On

My dad's health was declining rapidly, so Janet, Bryan and I flew down to Florida to see my parents. Pulling up to the gate of their condo, we announced ourselves and discovered that my parents weren't home. Crossing Jog Road into a strip mall, I drove toward the doctor's office and noticed my mother and father quietly walking slowly together toward their car. I found out later during our visit, that cancer had spread to his liver. My dad refused standard treatment and chose to live out the rest of his days with his wife in Delray Beach.

This may sound strange, but I can feel the relief – it's more than a reprieve, it's freeing, knowing the hardship that cancer carries within its core is suddenly removed. No more: "have tos," doctors' appointments, treatments, waiting for results and answers, wondering if what you do or don't do will affect its progress, hastening your departure.

How do I move from intellectualizing *I know I'm going to die, we all die at some point*, to internalizing, accepting it will happen, to embracing this most common human function? Do I have to wait until I learn it's imminent? I understand I haven't nuzzled up to this and I find it difficult to celebrate the ending. It's laced with sadness, loss, grief and my own anxieties. How to make peace with this?

For many years, I viewed my dad's decision to forgo treatment as one of the bravest things anyone could do. I still believe this, but also know that resigning to fate was part of my dad's character. Just as he demonstrated, when he realized my sister was different from other children, that she would need special care long after many of their friends' empty nests were built, my dad outwardly accepted this with open arms. He embraced Ronda with a loving heart. Now, after almost 11 years since the melanoma was discovered, numerous blood tests, doctor's visits, updates, explanations and hope, my dad surrendered to his reality.

With his ear-to-ear smiles, our 5-month-old son softened the air of sadness. It was a good visit, a time when Dad was still able to go out to dinner, take short walks and play rummy.

Taking turns pushing Bryan in his stroller, my dad and I took our last walk together. Not saying much, stepping over yellow painted speed bumps, we stopped to look at the shuffleboard courts and remembered playing here with Mom and Ronda. Pausing to watch people hit tennis balls over a net, it was obvious my dad was searching for the right words.

"You have to get over this."

"What do you mean?" I asked.

As my dad finished his next sentence, my immediate inclination was defensive and defiant, but recognizing our time was short, I internalized what I felt.

Three generations together: grandfather, father and son, traditions not yet established and few memories to fall back on, I began to feel the insignificance of so many things in life.

"You have to get over how you feel about Ronda."

While I erected unrealistic one-way mirrors, believing no one could see in, I was blinded by my own denial, yet I knew it was impossible to hide how I felt about Ronda. With thoughts of asking my dad what he meant, or saying things are different than he thinks, I decided in that moment to make and honor a commitment to look after my sister.

"Don't worry Dad, I'll take care of Ronda, I promise you."

When we arrived back home in Connecticut, time seemed to move rapidly. An early snowy winter melted into a premature spring.

APRIL 11, 1988

I would send books I thought my dad would enjoy, write letters or poetry and ask Mom to read certain excerpts as Dad's health declined. During conversations I'd listen to my mother's words and tone to gauge my dad's health, attempting to determine the best time to visit. Two months after our last visit, I left for Florida.

Dad didn't have the energy or desire to do much and stayed home most of the time. Thinner than a few months ago, his gaunt, fading color prevented me from moving closer. I tried to keep the shock of seeing him to myself. As I approached, I hesitated out of a similar concern I felt toward my sister – that I might catch what they had. At 7 years of age, once I believed my prayer would not be answered, I knew that I didn't want to identify with my sister's disabilities. I chose to hide behind my truth, creating masks that wouldn't let my authentic self emerge. I was distant. This identity crisis stayed with me for a very long time.

I made attempts, but repelled by my fears I found it hard to get physically close to my dad. Yet years before, after weeks in intensive care, with hope on the horizon, my father now sitting up in bed, I was more than willing and able to climb in with him, give him a shave, removing stubbles from his face, replacing them with jokes and talk of the future. It is possible to move beyond our self-imposed restrictions. And yet, it can be so difficult.

But now, seeing my dad at 73, my first parent close to the end of life, I didn't know how to act or react. For years, suppressing my emotions had been a full-time job. Fear turned to anger, irritation to hostility, disappointment to aggression and complacency. I'd worked hard to avoid revealing my emotions, refusing to allow them to surface or let my tears wash away sadness or fright, despair or heartache.

My dad and I sat together on the floral couch that was part of their turnkey $18,000 investment. White high-back wooden kitchen chairs, a small round dining table, matching glass cases on either side of the front door. Loveseat and ottoman all decorated in the same floral pattern. Their television centered against a wall in the living room. A small bedroom with twin beds, master bedroom to the right. A 4-foot by 10-foot sunroom facing the back, looking over the guest parking spot and my parents' space. My dad's white Chevrolet sat idle.

As we watched the NCAA basketball tournament, knowing in that moment we shared time and space and love for each other but little else, a distance like an invisible wedge existed between us. An attempt at playing cards brought little joy. As soon as I arrived, it felt like it was time to leave and there was not much to say. My dad was waiting. I already missed him.

Watching him sit in silence as he prepared to depart this life, knowing I would be leaving for Connecticut shortly, a rush of emotions turned to an overwhelming sense of isolation. A few days after saying hello, I said goodbye for the last time. A friend of my parents came to the front door to drive me to the airport.

"Have a nice life," my dad said as I stopped, turned and looked toward him.

The last time I would hear my dad's voice in person. He was a man of few words who primarily taught me by example, but these final four words of advice were profound and deeply saddening.

I walked to the bedroom leading to the sunporch and to their friend's car. Stoic and resolved to show little emotion, I left their condo. I didn't cry.

A few weeks later, my dad passed on.

SIX YEARS LATER I HEARD FROM MY DAD.

Eight-month-old Bryan was soon to have a baby brother. Strollers, baby walkers and swings, not much sleep, day care and nursery schools. Followed by "the shuttle service," driving our sons and their friends to and from soccer practice, T-ball games, after-school programs and birthday parties. On top of that, I was building a new career in business – so much to focus on and occupy my time for the next six years.

Feeling unsettled and incomplete since my father passed, when a healer said, "You can let go now," my world changed.

Strange things had been unfolding in our home. The clock radio in our bedroom repeatedly came on by itself. An upstairs television would spontaneously turn on, followed by the large TV in the living room. No patterns that I was aware of, just random occurrences. These unexplained phenomena took place a number of times, until I knew something beyond what I was capable of fully comprehending was happening – an unknown presence was in our lives.

Shortly after Bryan and Evan were born, I entered the foggy world of a "light sleeper" and was subjected to the nocturnal rustling, foraging and preying on those not so fortunate. Owls, coyotes, skunks finding their way around our backyard as night fell.

"What is that noise?" my coarse, startled voice woke Janet from a sound sleep. "Did you accidentally set the alarm for 2 a.m.?"

"No. I'll show you what time I set it for in the morning," Janet answered.

A few nights later I yelled in anger, "What is this? How did the TV turn on?"

Something, or someone, was trying to get our attention.

"I don't know," Janet said.

Looking at her, I replied, "I have an idea."

"Let's unplug the TVs before we leave for work today."

When we arrived home, we were astounded to hear music coming from the upstairs radio and a commercial promoting a sale from the still unplugged TV. We were continuously awakened from our sleep to late night shows or when the alarm tuned to a radio station set to come on at 6 a.m. decided 1:30 a.m. was a better time to wake us.

With intermittent help from therapists, I eventually came to realize that I had not been able to accept my father's passing, that it was possible my dad was hanging around to support me as I grieved in silence. Knowing how I struggled to be close to him toward the end of his life, I believed he was nudging me. Helping me along to let go and move to a better place, to be free and move on, carrying fond, loving memories.

A friend put me in touch with a spiritual healer. We talked by phone. This incredibly intuitive, compassionate woman recognized that I was not able or willing to say goodbye to my dad. Soft-spoken, easygoing, my dad whose whistling tune I heard four flights up as he entered the hallway to begin his climb from 12 hours of work to our small two-bedroom apartment. Happy to be home no matter the challenges awaiting him on the other side of the green door leading to apartment 3B or 4B. Of course, my father would try to let me know any way he could that he was here to help me. He appreciated my curiosity and acceptance of the spirit world and was guiding me. I was convinced he was making his presence felt.

Before our phone call ended, this wonderful healer concluded by saying "You can let go now." Moments later, hearing Janet, Bryan and Evan pulling into the driveway, I wiped my tears away. We all grieve in our own way and on our own time. I had done so by moving in and out of sadness, feeling glum or angry, distant or lonely but not crying. It took almost seven years after I lost my dad to cry. And yet, to this day, my long-standing stoic nature can get the best of me, preventing me from appearing vulnerable.

Two years later, as 9-year old Bryan slept in the second bedroom in my parents' condo, my father made another appearance. Startled and frightened, Bryan ran into the master bedroom and found Janet, Evan and me asleep in my parents' bed. "Grandpa Max! I saw Grandpa Max! He was here, he was looking at me!"

I understood and appreciated that my dad was now there for my mom as she approached the end of her battle with Parkinson's disease. Most of my mother's time during the last year before she moved to a nursing home was spent in the room Bryan was now staying in. As frightened as Bryan was, I was able to see the humor in this as well. The next morning I closed my eyes and appealed to my dad to stop coming over. "You must be confused, Mom is not living here anymore, she is staying at a nursing home a couple of miles away. You can visit her there."

From that time forward, my awareness of my dad has come in dreams or while awake recalling memories.

15

DO BUTTERFLIES CRY? ARE THEY MESSENGERS?

ugust 2003. A horseshoe of land protects and surrounds an inlet of gradual tides exposing sandbars and gentle waves. Here, the clear North Atlantic waters are insulated from the cold just a few miles away. By bike or walking through dunes to a wooden stairway extending toward a small boardwalk, a tucked away sign, its colors blending with white and tan shades of summer welcomes you to Crane Beach at Castle Hill on the North Shore of Massachusetts.

Perhaps from the constant movement of rocks over time, the sand is uniform, tiny pieces of gravel massage your feet while strolling along. Benches of driftwood find the shore at low tide, settling into the sand while geometric patterns form as water cuts and carves shapes that glisten in sunlight. Children play in collected pools of warm water. Bathers venture out to sandbars as the tide recedes. Dunes welcome tall grasses as plovers rustle to safety. Slender white birds with long necks dance along the shore of their namesake's beach.

Cool breezes found their way through an open restaurant window. A birthday eve dinner blended with good wishes for a successful interview. But what was planned as my 55th birthday celebration on the North Shore with my partner abruptly ended. A call from her soon-to-be-employer prompted Deborah to regretfully make arrangements to travel to Boston the next day.

As it should be toward the end of August, my birthday morning was clear, calm and pleasantly cool, no clouds to shroud the rising sun. It was a perfect day to fly. When I found myself walking to Crane Beach late morning, passing others with chairs, blankets, towels and coolers, slowly folding into my solitude, I began to feel peaceful.

Butterflies usually do not make their way to the ocean. It's rare to see one, yet on this day yellow, spotted wings softly fluttering, moving with purpose, keeping up with the ocean breezes, stayed close. As I turned, this delicate, graceful butterfly hovered, then flittered away as if a game, hiding, returning to join me as I sat on a long hollow sandalwood bench. Perched on my left shoulder, it sat as I pondered. When I rose, it hesitated, then launched, darted, paused and stayed with me as I sauntered back to my blanket and chair at the end of my stroll on this beautiful beach.

Something more than a walk with a new friend. Curiosity, an eerie sense of anticipation and surrender overwhelmed me. Finishing my lunch, I extended my chair, wrapped what was left of my sandwich, placed a colorful, striped beach towel under my head and fell into a restful midday nap. A while later, the sun now lower, shining over my left shoulder, reaching for the horizon, feeling slightly disoriented, I gradually opened my eyes and ears to the gentle sound of waves bringing in the tide and me back to life. Remembering the time spent with my friend I began looking and wondering again.

When I saw this butterfly on a towel under my beach chair, it appeared to be resting. Then I noticed its wings were still, sprawled, lifeless. When I placed my friend in my left hand a deep sense of sorrow filled me with a sadness that rushed through my body. As if I had lost someone close to me.

Warm, dry, late summer air stayed all day as I sat, read, napped or just watched people enjoying their time. A calm feeling comforted me as I carried this weightless insect to the shoreline. Within hours, what began as curiosity had moved to companionship, kinship, friendship and more. But it now resembled a burden, a personal loss. Praying for a moment, knee-deep clear, warm water surrounding me, I placed one of God's creatures to rest on a wave, watching for a while, and waiting as the tide carried it out to sea. I said goodbye for the first time. This day on Crane Beach would reveal its significance 16 months later

DECEMBER 3, 2004

As I always have, when I arrived home late weekday afternoons, pressing the remote to open the red-stained garage doors, I left my car carrying a briefcase, loose manila folders, and a box of 5x8 index cards (not containing customer names, dates and amounts owed, but school numbers, librarians names and directions). I walked up the stairs leading to the kitchen, then a bathroom stop on the way to my home office. Monday through Friday, this routine was the same. I wouldn't see my sons until dinner, when they would come home after their part-time jobs.

Now 17, Bryan's easy demeanor and soft, deliberate voice defined him. Similarities to Janet or myself weren't as obvious as they were when he was a baby. "Oh, he looks so like you," "He has your eyes, your hair," friends or strangers would freely comment. Dark hair similar in texture to mine, a reminder of my grandfather, Bryan wasn't built for long-distance running, unlike Evan and myself. But his strong legs provided the speed that served him well on the cross-country track teams in middle and high school.

Until he was 4, Evan's weight was well above the norm. So much so, that when he was 14 months old, his chunky arms concealed the veins needed to draw blood, making it impossible to test for Lyme Disease. (Fortunately, it didn't materialize.) Now 16, slender, his fine blonde hair falling toward his eyebrows having faded to light brown, my very personable, occasionally stubborn son loves the company of friends and family.

Tired and weary from driving for hours this second Friday in December, I pressed the play button on my answering machine after checking the fax for purchase orders. Three or four business messages, a pause, a sales call leading to another pause, I began settling into my desk chair.

A concerned voice from someone in Florida. "Something

has happened to your sister... perhaps falling into a deep sleep?"

In the recesses of my memory, to this day, I cannot find what else was said or if these were the exact words spoken. When I called the group home where my sister, 53, had been living in Fort Pierce, distressed, fearful, apologetic tones accompanied the story. "Ronda had choked on some food that afternoon while eating lunch in the workshop, a bus ride away from the group home. She is in the hospital. We don't know..." I tried to concentrate and listen, but I didn't want to or couldn't hear the rest. "Please tell me the number of the hospital and who to talk with."

Within seconds after saying I was Les Kalish, Ronda Kalish's brother, the head nurse in the ICU in Fort Pierce said, "Ronda is in a coma."

More about the incident was shared. But there were too many missing pieces, unknowns, not enough information to paint an accurate picture of what happened. Shocked and confused, I closed my eyes.

I have carried this haunting vision with me since that conversation. Perhaps Ronda was sitting alone, or with friends who didn't notice before it was too late that while eating a sandwich, some food had lodged in my sister's throat. Unable to speak, panic, fear, horror and then sorrow. Surrender carrying her along to the unknown. I don't want to imagine the minutes it must have taken my sister to yield, from when she couldn't swallow that bite of her sandwich to when she stopped trying to ask for help – when she moved from aware-ness to coma.

This is so unfair. Ronda: What you wanted most was to love and be loved. To spend time with people, enjoy their friendship, walk to town for pizza and a Coke, to help out in the kitchen. Unfair because the medication you were given to quell negative behavior, obstinance, outbursts or anger was an attempt to control you. Understandable, because without these stop gaps you couldn't live in the DeLeon group home. Otherwise you would be institutionalized. Mom, nor Dad, nor I would allow that to happen.

And so unfair because I suddenly realize I might not have a chance to make up for all the times I ignored, mistreated or resented you, walking out of your life. I feel so ashamed.

As that 7-year-old, not too long after I asked God to help you, something began to grow inside me. I was bewildered, then indignant. Doubts that God existed resurfaced and if he did, why didn't he hear me 49 years ago?

I resented that I had to carry this burden all these years and didn't get my wish, which was as much for me as it was for you. Disappointed and feeling powerless, I didn't know if I still had a chance to care for and look after you. Thank you, God, for taking my parents before this happened. Reality coalesced with relief.

Faced with my sister's health crisis, my thoughts returned to my parents' passings. During the last visit with my dad, I'd felt as though I was staring at death and I was horrified. Mom had called me the morning after Dad passed on in their bed. She was grateful for friends who rushed over to help and her sighs mixed with tears of grief signaled that she was beginning a new journey, more alone in the world as my father's voyage came to an end and a new one began. As much as I loved my dad, I was relieved not to be there when he died.

Not quite 10 years after my father passed, before Parkinson's took its toll on my mother, I was hoping to be with her at the end. Time changed what felt like a reluctant responsibility to a desire. My mom was alone, and I wanted her to know I was there.

Mom, just days away from leaving this earth, after years of attempting to befriend Parkinson's disease, I was reminded of your resilience, positive attitude and love of reading and writing. As evidenced in the many abbreviated cards and letters you had sent, your handwriting painted a picture of your struggles. The last day I saw you in person, moving closer, talking loudly so you could hear my attempts to comfort you, the words you uttered had stunned me. "I don't want to go."

Distance and predictability made it virtually impossible to spend large blocks of time with you in Florida toward the end of your life, and regretfully I was not there when you passed on.

"Can you book me a flight out of Bradley to Florida? The hospital called; they think my mother is nearing the end." Janet bought me a seat on the 8 p.m. flight to Fort Lauderdale. By the time I arrived at the hospital at Del Ray Beach, it was nearly 1 a.m.

Sitting in a chair beside my mother's bed, holding her hand, I noticed her peaceful, relaxed expressions as she slept. I had to focus on her shallow breaths, the gradual rise and fall of her gown to see if she was still with us. To my surprise, we both woke up in the early morning.

I wasn't disappointed but I didn't anticipate this. Yesterday's conversation with the head nurse still fresh in my mind prepared me to be greeted with the news that Mom had passed. Now, after a few hours of sleep, my palm moist, my hand stiff, her doctor told me that Mom will be moved to a shared room to rest with hopes of returning to the nursing home in a few days. I flew home the next afternoon.

Entering the parlor at the I.J. Morris Funeral Home on Long Island for Mom's service, cousin Melvin stopped me. It had been a long time since we last saw each other.

"Your mother did a wonderful job with Ronda."

"I appreciate your kind words. Thanks Mel."

"I was aware of my mom's personal struggles, the challenges and hardships of raising a daughter with special needs in the 1950s. I was also mindful of her strength and resolve, and timeless efforts to help Ronda approach her potential." I spoke these words at the beginning of my eulogy for Edith Kalish on March 19, 2002, six days after I returned from seeing her in Florida. Mom was 85. Her fear of dying young, like her mother, had not materialized.

I HAD LITTLE TIME OR DESIRE TO REFLECT YET FELT forced to stop and reconnect. Sitting on our white and blue speckled sofa, its back resting on the gold metal strip that finished off the fading gray carpet dividing my office and its hardwood floors from the TV room, I closed my eyes. Attempting to stay calm, bringing myself back to where I sat 20 years before, learning to meditate, asking for guidance, a vision appeared. Focusing on my sister, I began to see images of a smooth, white oval form and tried to make sense of it.

Praying intently and asking for a miracle, I eventually resigned myself to the worst possible outcome. I regretted that I couldn't change anything about my day that would have prevented this from happening, so I continued to pray and ask for help.

Pacing around my office in shock, knowing I couldn't turn to my mother or father anymore, I knew I had to fly to Florida. Bryan and Evan went to their mom's. Who else do I ask for help?

While there were many times I felt alone throughout my life, I always had a sense that I was looked after. When flying down to the nursing home or hospital as Parkinson's aged with my mother, I was accompanied by an unknown but undeniable presence – angels. They appeared in dreams or as a white speck in the rearview mirror of my car, floating but not there. I have been able to tune in and out of a low frequency, clearly telling me that I wasn't alone, a calming presence in the midst of turbulence. I have felt as though I can rely on something beyond our worldly existence to guide me or just to be there, keeping me company. I was and continue to be grateful.

Pierce, conversations with the group home staff, doctors and nurses all trying to make sense of what happened, what to expect and what to do next consumed much of my time; quiet contemplation, searching for answers while meditating under a tree, running to keep my head clear. Hours and hours, long days and nights in the ICU.

Other families sat and waited for their own answers,

hoping and praying for their loved ones. I sought counseling from clergy, looked for guidance as I was the one ultimately responsible for taking Ronda off life support, and prayed for confirmation that my visions of my sister already joining my parents were accurate.

I hoped I would be able to move past feeling responsible for my sister's passing. That I could let go of guilt. Not just what I felt growing up in Bensonhurst, but as a young man living on my own, making little effort to see Ronda, and as an adult busy with my own children, too occupied to reach out. But also giving into the reality that I didn't have the ability or the power to prevent this unspeakable tragedy from happening. Where are you God?

16

TAKING A RISK, DISAPPOINTMENT, CONFIRMATION

Originally a Jesuit seminary, Kripalu in Lenox, Massachusetts, was more than a getaway for me. It was a place to reconnect to my spirituality, to heal, practice yoga and meditate. Find like-minded seekers, hike through the Berkshires and eat food prepared the way I prefer but didn't often take the time to do so.

Three months before my 55th birthday and four months away from being divorced, Kripalu felt like a safe place to attend an intensive weekend program designed to connect spiritual seekers. I was also hoping to meet someone to share time with. When I walked into the room Friday night, I noticed a woman sitting toward the center on the floor by herself. Within minutes of joining her, I strongly felt and believed that we were placed together for a reason. It's certainly possible that the circumstances surrounding me, affected what I sensed. I was moving through a divorce, raising two teenagers, attempting to reconnect to my spirituality and cautiously craving a healthy relationship. But there was more.

Among the many things I temporarily lost sight of during 18 years of marriage was how to freely enter into a relationship with confidence – that taking a risk would lead to opening my heart again.

As Deborah and I talked, sharing stories before the program began, some personal, some not, I knew there was something familiar about us. I sat on the floor with Deborah throughout this introductory class and became aware of signs and messages from outside of myself. They were subtle, leading me to new discoveries, but one was clear and obvious, and very familiar.

As the room filled, she began to tell me about her children. Deborah's daughter was living with her in Massachusetts attending high school and her son, who is on the autism spectrum, spent time between his dad's and mom's. Ronda was living at DeLeon House in Florida and I was overseeing her care from another state, believing I was fulfilling the promise I had made to my dad. So drawn in by the story of her son, I moved close to a woman I had just met and attached two invisible lures as an old tape replayed itself.

Here I go again.

Another opportunity to make things right – take what I've learned and have been carrying with me my whole life, and to be there for someone I know I can help. Gaining Deborah's love and approval, another chance to heal old relationships. A light in the midst of turmoil and heartbreak as my marriage faded. Hope. In the short time it took these thoughts and feelings to stir within me, I also recognized that this would be challenging and potentially heartbreaking.

Walking Deborah to her car that Sunday, after the long weekend, I knew from now on a day would not pass without thinking about her. A few weeks later, midway between Central Massachusetts and New Milford, Connecticut, Deborah and I pulled into a Park and Ride in separate cars. We left in my car making our way down a remote, winding road. No destination, no plan, just spending time. "We're keeping company." Stopping the car, turning toward Deborah, I asked her where she'd heard that. Along with those words and her response, "I don't know, but I felt compelled in that moment to say that," confirmed what I believed I knew on the floor at Kripalu two weeks before. Soft, joyful tears slowly found my cheeks. In that moment, I felt as though my mother was giving us her blessing.

I hadn't heard that phrase, "keeping company" since I was a young boy. Words spoken in conversations between aunts and uncles, parents and grandparents describing a family member who is beyond dating and moving into a serious relationship. "Keeping company," these sweet words were always greeted with "oohs" and "aahs" and smiles unless, of course, the boy or girl wasn't Jewish.

A few days before taking my sister off life support, I called Deborah, then my partner of a year-and-a-half. Appreciating the hardships she faced with her son, and being protective by nature, I shared only pieces of this frightful experience my sister and I were facing during the times Deborah and I spoke on the phone. "Sadly," I said, "I have decided to take Ronda off life support." This was so hard to say on many levels.

I was hardly one to ask for help. But I did so because my sister's life was in my hands. Having made the decision to remove all support was too much to bear alone – so I took a chance.

Just uttering those words aloud, "take Ronda off life support" confirmed my decision. I dreaded her response, knowing that what Deborah was about to say could define our relationship from this time forward. "Will you come down to Florida and be with me?"

"I can't. I can't do that," Deborah sadly but firmly answered.

The woman I loved, who'd pulled at my heartstrings until tender music pried it open again, broke it. We hung up.

Saying Goodbye Again

Staff members gathered with me, surrounding Ronda as she lay in her bed on the fifth floor in the ICU. With fresh visions of dreams, possible scenarios laid out by nurses and likely outcomes, a surprisingly lighthearted exchange surfaced as the director of DeLeon House, aides and other support staff shared stories. Stories with a theme: how much Ronda enjoyed dancing, which boyfriend she would choose on a given night, how certain she could be of anything – reminders of our mother.

"She loved to eat. It didn't matter what was prepared, she

was always hungry," a staff member shared. We all laughed in agreement.

"She was such a social person. On the dance floor Ronda would freely join in," another aide said holding back tears while smiling. "She just loved to be around people."

Stories continued. My sister's love of music, being with friends, and how much she missed her mom, dad, and her brother.

I'm right here Ronda, I'm right here.

How drawn she was to animals, how often she would tell staff they were doing something incorrectly, how observant she could be. Twenty years after I began growing my beard, the time felt right for a new look. Clean shaven, only Ronda commented. It was the first thing she said when we saw each other. "Les, you shaved. I like it."

As my stress level was rising, the stories faded. It was eerie, like a ceremony was about to take place. The room grew quiet and we were led in prayer. The most vivid image I had of my sister not breathing when all the tubes and respirator were removed, did not happen. To my surprise and relief, Ronda was breathing effortlessly. A ray of hope surfaced. But, before I concluded that we'd witnessed a miracle, the head nurse explained that even after five days on life-support and no brain activity, Ronda could continue to breathe on her own and may do so for a while.

The comfort of now familiar faces diminished. The day wore on until I found myself alone in a private room watch-fully waiting for something to happen. Little did I know a similar phrase (watchful waiting) would be so meaningful to me in a different way, later in life. A long night in and out of sleep in a chair next to Ronda's bed turned to morning. Because she was still breathing on her own, preparations were made to transport her to hospice. Everything happened so fast.

Now in the back of an ambulance together, we turned off the main road and entered a long parking lot surrounded by evergreens. Then a hush, as if God sighed. An oasis appeared out of nowhere, silence so loud it calmed every cell in my body. The cacophony of emotions suddenly ended.

Approaching a house with an inviting front porch, the ambulance slowed down then came to a stop. I followed the driver's lead and left my sister. Immediately, but calmly, I was greeted at the porch. "Please give us a little time to get your sister settled in." A shroud of tranquility, an inviting quiet environment washed away six days of horror as trauma, shock and sadness turned into a peaceful reality.

Robin, the supervisor of my sister's group home, and I stood outside waiting to be called. Gazing overhead, I noticed a group of hawks hovering. Many times, while sitting on a bench or in the grass at the grounds of the hospital this long week, as time seemed to stand still, I had noticed hawks searching for thermals to glide on. It was as though they were gathering for something. I concluded that hawks were messengers waiting to transport newly departed souls. This helped guide me as I surrendered to our fate. My part of this journey was almost over.

December 10, 2004

It was a calm, warm, comfortably humid evening in Fort

Pierce, Florida. I would stay the night with Ronda then fly home in the morning. My sister was lying comfortably in her bed, no bars, breathing tubes, charts or monitors. A few staff members from the DeLeon home were still with her.

As the afternoon waned, I reluctantly agreed to take the drive with Robin to the group home to gather Ronda's personal belongings. It was clear to everyone that Ronda's time was very close to the end – I so desperately wanted to be there.

I was hesitant to leave my sister because I wanted to be with her when it was her time. I was the only one left with the same blood passing through our veins. I had a promise to keep and I wanted to fulfill it.

Feeling rushed at the group home, we gathered Ronda's personal items then drove back to hospice. As we pulled into the parking lot, I was resigned to leave the next day. Closing the car door, I looked toward the porch and noticed arms waving in our direction, beckoning us. Walking faster, now almost running, a nurse shuttled us into Ronda's room. Some words were spoken about an "ending" as we all gathered around. Laboring, my sister let go of her final breath.

As the shadows of my sister's afterlife hovered, I could clearly see my mother sculpt herself, morphing within Ronda. Not just visions in my mind's eye but a truly remarkable transformation. My mother welcoming her daughter, blessing her with wisdom, guiding her through this transition, still teaching. Stunned, no thoughts, I wailed, crying deeply for my sister Ronda, as I said goodbye, not quite a year-and-a-half later, for the second time.

My fragile, yellow-spotted winged friend was close in thought.

She waited for me. Ronda knew I wanted to be there and showed me how to let go and move on. Throughout her life, my sister gave me the most beautiful gift, her unconditional love. "I hope I can repay you in the next life. I love you."

When filling out my sister's death certificate, rather than leave occupation blank I wrote "social worker."

ATTEMPTING TO LISTEN

Sometimes free will is not all it's cracked up to be. It's almost impossible to do what you know in your heart is in your best interest especially when that same heart pleads for you to stay.

Deborah and I made concessions surrounding unspoken doubts. We knew we were entering dangerous waters, but we continued our search. Numerous days with a realtor, frustration and doubt surfaced, so I asked the universe for guidance. "Please show us the house we're looking for."

Six months after my sister passed, eleven days before her 55th birthday, Deborah and I celebrated two years of keeping company and moved into a home, perched on the crest of a steep hill in East Greenwich, Rhode Island. You can get what you want but not necessarily what you need.

Making peace with Ronda's passing, grieving over time, my sister's memory brightened. But things with Deborah dimmed. The more Deborah's son stayed with us, the clearer it became that I wasn't willing to play a role in this all too familiar drama. There was nothing for me to prove, no karmic debts to repay. I didn't feel obligated to myself or to Deborah to continue supporting her through the tumultuous relationship with her son. I also felt a sense of completion when she considered working for the Autism Foundation. As my mother had, Deborah recognized her strengths and the value of her personal experiences. She found herself at a time in her life when the important work she was here to do had arrived and I took pride and satisfaction in knowing that I was able to help guide her toward that realization.

Shortly after Deborah's dad passed on, to get away, perhaps start fresh, to remember and let go, we decided to book a whitewater rafting trip down the Middle Fork of the Salmon River in Idaho. Sitting across from Deborah in our six-person raft, I spotted an orange and black butterfly hovering overhead. Seconds later it moved toward Deborah. We were drifting, the butterfly moving in and out of sight. It was a quick visit but just long enough for me to remember my birthday on Crane Beach and my sister.

The third day on the river, our colorful friend reappeared, joining us for a ride. It would leave, then return minutes or hours later. We both felt that Deborah's dad was present. Perhaps resting on a leaf at night, each morning this butterfly would happily reintroduce itself until our final day on the river. With a flick and flutter, hovering then playfully darting away, our friend kept us company. On the sixth day, regretfully accepting the void once we realized this beautiful creature wasn't coming back, life began to brighten for Deborah.

A bout with pneumonia, little approval from my children

and struggles with my business were taking their toll on our relationship.

Five years felt like a moment. The summer of 2008 arrived early in Rhode Island and mid-June felt like late July. My sons were on their way to our house for the weekend. I reserved three kayaks for Saturday. We would paddle along the bay, stop for lunch stowed away in our backpacks, take a break and talk.

Driving to the boat launch I began to feel lightheaded. Leaving our car, walking to the shore, I began to feel ashamed. It felt like a brief flash of time. I was embarrassed to tell anyone that Deborah and I were ending our relationship, especially my children, and that their father was going through another breakup so soon after the divorce. What I didn't share with them were the reasons I was so deeply hurt – that my heart had healed five years ago and now ached again in ways I didn't want to remember.

Five years after my divorce, it felt as though I was living through it again. However, this time was different. No financial documents or commitments to divide, only some furniture and a few plants. But still, how to reconcile and move past the pain? What I did let Bryan and Evan know was how much I looked forward to spending more time with them because I was moving into a condo in Old Lyme, Connecticut. "We will be in the same state again," I said with assurance. What I didn't know was that the next five years of my life would present challenges I had hoped and worked so hard to avoid.

It's never too late to apologize. Children are often put in a position to divide loyalties, choose one parent over another or accept a parent's new partner unquestionably. Just because their mom or dad finds happiness or now seems lighter as the dark shadows of their marriage begin to brighten, doesn't completely erase any confusion or resentment children may carry.

Perhaps my sons are stronger because of what we all went through and maybe scars of lost opportunities are fading. Consumed by hurt, uncertainty, living in a void makes it difficult to be present not only for yourself but for others. *I deeply regret not being more available as my marriage dissolved and for exposing you to my painful breakup.*

BACK IN CONNECTICUT ON MY OWN, MY FEELINGS difficult to conceal, depressed at times, often melancholy, my sorrow punctuated my masks. I moved through my days as authentically as any other time in my life. These feelings were all too familiar. An elderly neighbor, librarians on business calls, friends and my children recognized what I felt and in their own way tried to be supportive.

Yoga was now an important part of my life. Running for 25 years, primarily on pavement, had taken its toll. Attempts to replace it with biking, searching for the elusive runner's high were unsuccessful. Yoga filled some of the gaps, offering a calming as I stretched my body into and out of asanas, learning some of the subtleties of Iyengar, Ashtanga and Hatha yoga. I spent many days after work, sometimes Saturdays, at a studio practicing a relatively new form of yoga, Svaroopa, appreciating many of the contemplative free-flowing poses and accompanying meditations. This evolved into a small community of like-minded people, including a friend a few years older than me, who had recently embarked on a journey that I would soon join.

I WAS STILL SEARCHING WHEN I UNEXPECTEDLY FOUND what soothes my soul, and just maybe a glimpse of what I was looking for all these years.

I decided to enroll in a weeklong intensive training at Kripalu to enhance my yoga practice. Kripalu has always been a source of awakenings and new beginnings. With the excitement of this adventure in front of me, I drove to the Berkshires as spring anticipated summer's arrival.

Perhaps stress, my age now 59, and grief combined, were taking their toll as many of my poses were more difficult to hold than they had been five years earlier. Arching my back while in warrior one was a challenge, and a simple seated forward bend brought me virtually half as close to my outstretched legs. Bowing in child's pose was still soothing, as was lying in shavasana's resting pose when ending a session. Simply existing with my eyes closed. No thoughts. Just being.

I sought out Swami Nirmalananda, the founder of Svaroopa yoga, who was leading this program, at the end of a morning session to ask about some postures. My hidden agenda was counsel for an aching heart. Nearly 6 feet tall, short cropped hair showing early signs of gray, Swami's placid facial expression and calming eyes were alluring. At her request, I found myself lying face down on a yoga mat in half frog.

Recognizing my uneasiness, Swami Nirmalananda said to

me as she carefully adjusted my lower back, her hands awakening something within me, "You know this is emotional?"

I lay there for a minute or so. Saddened, I looked back at her in agreement.

As soon as I reached the back of the room, opening the palatial doors leading to the main hallway, an uncontrollable rush to purge something so deep inside overtook me. Fearing I would throw up, pass out, or who knows what, I began to run faster and faster, hoping to get to my room in time. A few long breaths sitting on my bed, years of deep sadness, grief and heartache washed through me, not just recent losses, but what felt like old hurts and ancient traumas as well. I was crying for more than just myself.

As sighs of relief finally brought me back to earth, I couldn't remember a time in my life when I felt so at peace. I walked back down the narrow hallway to the cafeteria knowing I was surrounded by only what was right in the world, all along feeling connected to energies outside my earthly body.

Sitting with Swami a few days later, describing my experience, I asked if I could realistically expect to walk through the rest of my life like this.

"It's possible but impractical. You're meant to be here on earth and do the work you came to do. You may find this again later in life, or in another life," Swami Nirmalananda explained in a soft, comforting tone.

I wanted to hold onto this as long as possible. I don't have to imagine; I knew what it is to be judgment free, welcoming with an open heart, and privy to an approaching moment while living in the present one. To want for nothing more than what I have. I was one with the universe and knew God existed within me.

By the next day's lunch, the intensity of these feelings was already fading. Yet, they were still strong enough to carry me through the remainder of this week. I didn't know it then, but what I discovered at Kripalu may have been what I was searching for all these years.

BACK HOME WHILE SITTING IN LOTUS POSITION, I VIEWED the blueprint of my life so far. My takeaway, what I firmly believed, is that my spiritual awareness can lead me to endless possibilities. What was I taught when I was a young boy, asking God for a miracle? Perhaps patience, and later in life that my sister was here to teach me kindness, unconditional love, sacrifice and so much more. That 7-year-old boy's wish wasn't meant to be answered, at least, not as I had hoped. There was a bigger plan.

What did I learn when I was spared from witnessing Little Tim's tragic accident, my innocence preserved a while longer, my imagination creating scenes that would appear in nightmares as a child? Gratitude.

I was given the gift of appreciation and love. Soon after we met as teenagers, Steve, whose mere presence, no matter how far apart or for how long we lost contact, has guided and supported me through this life's journey. I know he feels the same.

Thankfulness for the lingering sense that I was always looked after, no matter how lonely I may have felt or isolated I may have been.

Have I benefited from these blessings, the difficult lessons I have learned as well as the delightful times spent with others? Most definitely.

In meditations as I awaited confirmation that there is indeed more. Time spent with healers actually seeing what I had only been able to sense.

What gift was I given when taken away in a dream to an extraordinarily bright light, revealing family members awaiting my mother's arrival just two days before she passed on? The awareness that it was indeed her time and she was being looked after.

The gifts of butterflies, causing me to pause, move inward and emerge in wonderment and peace.

Is our learning more significant the deeper the wound, or the more profound our experiences may be in life? Sometimes a traumatic experience or spiritual awakening – loss or major disruption can give us opportunities to reflect and go where we infrequently find ourselves. It can be the impetus to make drastic changes. Whatever it may be that puts a halt to life as we knew it might have a lasting impact, but more than likely will become a distant memory. Human nature being what it is will often take us back to where and who we were before. And to how we viewed, reacted and internalized the world, as we continue walking through our days to a familiar beat.

To this point in my life I knew much about myself but couldn't connect all the dots. I don't believe I was meant to bridge the gaps, like weaving significance in those poignant times, making it possible to remain present in the light. I wasn't ready.

. . .

Back home at a studio, evening yoga classes were not just about escaping the day, feeling my body breathe again, calming my mind. They grew into a social gathering and Sam and I were at the center. A tall, gregarious, outgoing man with a commanding voice, Sam stood out. Seeking clarity for a posture or just wanting to comment during every class, it was hard to miss Sam. This Svaroopa yoga class was our first shared experience.

As I approached 60, a series of blood tests for life insurance and an annual physical revealed a slowly rising PSA (prostate specific antigen). With complete faith in Sherry, a naturopathic intuitive, practicing in Bridgeport, CT, I relied on her instincts and medical background to guide me. A well-educated alternative practitioner in her mid-40s, she is a throwback to a previous generation and connected to other-worldly energies. The next two years brought with them fluctuations in PSA levels; 0.2, 0.8, 0.4, 1.2, 0.9, 1.6. I learned that 0 to 4.0 is considered a safe zone, but a rising PSA can be suspicious. Each visit to Sherry's office confirmed there was no need to worry. "Your prostate is not concerned," Sherry often said while closing her eyes as she sought guidance.

I had brought my children to Sherry since they were young boys and have been a patient for over 20 years. Her ability to read my physical, emotional and spiritual patterns was extraordinary. A variety of supplements modified during each appointment, diet, and encouragement to go within, listen and meditate were the prescriptions she shared. I often found the last part of the script difficult to adhere to. On my own, working as hard as I ever had, I made little time to explore my spirituality, except for yoga. My mother's anticipated destiny at 56, my father's cancer diagnosis at 62, and here I was now about to turn 60.

My friend Sam was nearing the end of a social work career. He was struggling with the desire to be closer to his daughters living in California, and his wife's wish to live near her children and young grandchildren in Connecticut. When we first met, I didn't know Sam had a biopsy a year or so earlier to determine if prostate cancer was present.

Facing these issues that were complicating Sam's life understandably prevented him from being available to foster a close friendship. Even so, we spent some time talking about what he had been through, including finding a urologist he felt he could trust, his feelings about biopsies, always comparing PSA levels and just getting to know each other better. Months before Sam's divorce and move to the west coast, I believe he was facing potentially serious decisions. I was not yet there and felt strongly that I wouldn't be considering doing anything but perhaps watchful waiting for the rest of my life.

Not too long after Sam and I met, I received a call from an old friend Phil who worked with one of the publishers I represented. Before we began talking about business, he explained how important it was for him to see his young children grow into adults. He believed his best option to witness this was to have prostate surgery. My friend was 51 at the time.

Looking forward to my 60th birthday, toward the end of the summer, I found myself walking along the beach in Watch Hill, Rhode Island, gearing up for my busy fall season, when my cell phone rang. John, who had his own consulting business, and I were friendly competitors. He needed someone to talk to. I learned he had been treated for prostate cancer a year ago and elected not to have surgery. He wanted to share his experience with the lingering side effects of his treatment.

Like it or not, guided by my own journey, learning that my friends were struggling with prostate cancer, my curiosity piqued. I began to learn more about this disease. Before Sam moved to California, he had a second and third biopsy. Cancer was detected during the second one but not the third. I became aware of conflicting information about the thoroughness as well as potential side effects of biopsies. Samples from the entire prostate cannot be taken. In addition, there is a possibility of infection and if there is cancer, it can spread during the biopsy. I also learned that much has been written about the validity of stand-alone PSA blood tests.

18

LOOKING FOR SIGNS, A KISS
SEALS IT

Can that actually be her? I thought to myself while driving through the parking lot to the restaurant. *I hope not!*

I approached a woman who was leaning on the top railing leading to the front door. A vague but distant resemblance to the picture posted on the dating website took me by surprise. How could someone age 20 years overnight? I helped her up the stairs, and to our table wondering why anyone would misrepresent themselves in this way.

This, and a series of eventful but unsuitable matches shortly after I turned 60 left me considering that I might walk through the rest of my life without a partner to share my heart with. As disturbing as that seemed, my online dating experiences made a good case for yielding to this possibility. I was beginning to believe arranged marriages were a good idea. Of course, I was 40 or so years too late and perhaps living in the wrong country.

Give it one more try. I didn't follow some of the advice eHarmony posted leading up to our initial meeting. Coffee or drink, not dinner; meet in a public place; don't drive together.

Mary suggested we meet for dinner in New Haven. We had moved beyond responding to online questions and emails to talking on the phone. Traveling from a conference in Philadelphia by train back to Boston, Mary would get off in New Haven, where I would pick her up. We would have dinner at an Italian restaurant not too far away. Nothing like listening to advice, really!

A confident, strong, beautiful woman approached. As Mary crossed the street from the train station and walked toward my car, lifelong impressions began to take shape. A firm handshake, engaging brown eyes and a warm, ready smile accompanied laughter. This assured, attractive woman was determined.

"Are you an ax murderer?" was her question after "Hi, how are you? I'm Mary."

I placed her suitcase in the trunk of my CRV, opened the passenger door, then replied as we turned to face each other, "I gave that up a few years ago."

Warm laughs melted the ice as questions about her trip and work followed. No awkward moments of silence. Anticipation calmed as excitement grew. The short ride to Basta was filled with conversation.

Both on the way to and from the restroom, Mary made a point to speak to our dinner neighbors – revealing confidence, kindness and a desire to be with people. However, still no clear sign from the universe that this was destiny, but also no need to text Evan, my backup ready to get me out of this date.

Walking around a nearby park before Mary's train arrived to take her back to Boston, I was still looking for signs. On the platform, crossing the threshold to her waiting train and to our lives, all the confirmation I needed found me as we kissed for the second time.

On her way home we talked for hours. From a chair in my condo, I spoke with Mary as her train moved north through Connecticut, passing Old Lyme, the town we would eventually live in together for two years. Her train continued through New London, home of Connecticut College, attended by Mary and then her daughter Ellie.

When I met Ellie a few weeks later, she had recently returned from a semester abroad in Argentina. As we sat outside on their back deck enjoying lunch, I learned about Ellie's time away, what her summer plans were and saw how forthright and generous she can be. Her curiosity allowed me to share more about myself.

Four weeks after we met, planning dinner, cleaning the condo, feeling light and excited, I anticipated Mary's arrival at the Old Saybrook station on Friday afternoon. No headboard on my bed, so I bought one – just in case. We spent time together a few weeks before in Rhode Island and many hours on the phone in between. Our budding relationship was unfolding in a beautiful way.

Four-and-a-half months later, we moved in together and Mary's occasional commute to New York City was virtually cut in half. When the last piece of furniture found a home, Bryan and Evan, Mary and I celebrated over dinner at a local restaurant. Arriving back at the condo, greeted by Arrow,

Mary's golden retriever, and her cats, this 1,800-square-foot, two-story abode suddenly felt different. A new energy permeated wood floors and stairs, glass and soon to be repainted walls. Warm touches, cloth napkins replacing paper towels, cut colorful flowers and indoor ferns, candles and new music.

Not too long after we met, Mary invited her son to join us at her family's house on the Cape for the weekend. Robbie's outgoing personality is hard to miss.

"Sit down over here at the dining table," Robbie requested.

As we sat across from each other, Robbie's question didn't surprise me. Being protective of his Mom he asked, "What are your intentions with my mother?"

"Only good," I replied.

Robbie pressed on. "Do you remember what she was wearing when you first met?"

"I can't recall how she was dressed," I added with a serious look and a hint of a smile. "I only remember gazing into her warm, brown eyes as we talked and shared our dinner."

We quickly moved onto other topics, as we continued to get to know each other.

I shared my concerns with Mary surrounding what I was learning about prostate cancer, my father's journey, and what some of my friends were facing. Her unconcerned look matched her words. "I'm not worried. Together we will face this and whatever finds us." At first, I found it difficult to accept that someone would be there for me. Mary's response opened a door, one that led me to a place I had not spent much time in as an adult or child and began to unlock my heart again. For so long, on many levels, I felt as though I was a reluctant caretaker, or in a relationship that fed my desire to be in charge or in control. *Now I can yield, let down my guard.*

I also broached our almost seven-year age difference. Both August birthdays, I was born a year after Israel was declared its own state and shortly before Bobby Thompson hit the home run against the Dodgers' Ralph Branca, "The shot heard round the world." Mary came into the world seven years after me, during Dwight D. Eisenhower's presidency and the 84th Congress, the debut of CBS TV's "To Tell the Truth" and 11 years into the Cold War.

"Our age difference doesn't bother me. I like you for who you are."

I did embrace Mary's sentiments and knew beyond any doubt that as I am for her, Mary is there for me.

A YEAR AWAY FROM 62, MY ANXIETIES CONTINUED TO increase as blood was drawn, searching for imbalances and measuring my PSA levels. PSA numbers remained under 4 and no evidence to cause concern except for a changing urgency to urinate that interrupted dreams. Even so, I became preoccupied, noting how many times I rose at night, how much water I drank each day and if that might impact a phone appointment or my drive. I was alert to different symptoms and continued to educate myself more and more.

The actual drawing of blood has never been a problem for me, but the time between, deciding when to do so and when I walked into Quest Diagnostics, made me anxious. Whether a few weeks or months, as that day approached uncertainty grew into uneasiness, then to a subtle anxiety that slowly surfaced, intensifying as the time drew near.

Purposeful days directed by routines and filled with meetings absorbed much of my time. A glass of wine with dinner eased my mind. Still the "ticker" – an unconscious stream of thoughts – was relentless. This fed concerns for my health, deeply rooted in my mother's beliefs and my father's illness.

THE RIGHT MOMENT

A year after we met, I was thrilled to discover Robert, Mary's father would be with us down the Cape the third weekend in May. A tall renaissance man, dapper and confident, he was more than willing to spin a tale and share his opinion. Always searching for ways to help; a true gentleman. Born in Pennsylvania, an ardent Cubs fan, he became a devoted Red Sox fan and raised his only child, to appreciate and love baseball. He was facing open heart surgery and my window to speak with him was closing.

Robert and his wife, Irene, who warmly welcomed me into their family, had lived a mile from Mary's Cape house for years before moving to a retirement community not too long before Mary and I met. Their love of friends, pine, oak and locust trees speckled in lichen, salty air filled with North Atlantic breezes still fresh in their hearts, often brought them back. Irene's charming, curious nature is contagious. Her concern for everyone she knows matches her eagerness to assist anyone in need.

When Mary left Saturday afternoon to run errands, I invited Robert to sit at the dining room table and asked for his permission to marry his daughter.

"I think that's a good idea," Robert said, pleased.

"I am working with a jeweler designing a ring I think Mary will like. I wanted to ask you now, before your surgery, but please don't tell anyone. Not even Irene."

"Oh, that makes a lot of sense," Robert laughed. "Where will you get married, and when?"

"Well, we haven't talked about this, but you know Mary. Once I propose, I'm sure she'll have a few ideas. We know how much Mary loves to plan," I pointed out.

We both chuckled.

Much of Mary's work at the time centered around organizing and implementing meetings, bringing together people from diverse sectors, uncovering their commonalities. And she loves to plan our dinners, vacations, outings with friends, family get-togethers. Her affable, outgoing nature mirrors her dad's.

Our conversation turned to a cup of tea and the newspaper for Robert, office work for me.

If I share something I believe will penetrate my mask do you now see me in a different light? Will you think less of me? I firmly believed I was okay, but doubts persisted. Not wanting to overburden Mary, create undue concern, appear weak or influence her perception of me, at times I hesitated to bring her into many of my private moments. Old habits were still hard to break.

I convinced myself that if I had prostate cancer, what I was learning positioned me with most men who wouldn't be adversely affected by this disease. Most of us will live with an enlarged prostate and it's not uncommon for PSA levels to rise after 60 years of age. Fluctuations can be caused by a number of variables and upwards of 85 percent of men who live into their 80s will have prostate cancer and most of them may not have to do anything about it.

Even so, the last three years, when anticipating time off as my busy work season came to a close, the breath of relief became less and less pronounced. My dwindling passion for my business and an emerging anxious eye on my health concerns, battled for my attention.

When I picked up the engagement ring at the jeweler, what I'd designed was more beautiful than I'd imagined. A few days later, as I opened a bottle of champagne, dinner just about prepared and ready to plate, I asked Mary to join me in the dining room. Pausing before we began, I excused myself. Arriving with a rather large box, I explained that I was sorry for being crabby lately and asked Mary to open her present. With a delightfully surprised look, Mary began to open a large box leading to a smaller one, then another and finally the tiniest, all beautifully wrapped.

Building anticipation culminated in tears of pure joy, ring

in hand, and "Yes" as I asked Mary to be my wife. A few moments later, I asked Mary another potentially life-changing question. Mary continues to go to a Protestant church. I haven't been inside a synagogue for years.

"Will you convert?" I asked, while in a tender embrace.

With a slight squint but peering directly into my eyes, Mary confidently replied, "I will never be a Yankees fan!"

Pleased that she wasn't easily persuaded; a sure sign of strength, character and loyalty, our heated rivalry remained intact. "And I will never become a Boston Red Sox fan," I replied. You can bet the house on that!

We spent much free time planning our early fall wedding. I found myself working outside planting trees and shrubs, expanding my vegetable garden, painting parts of the house, creating an even more welcoming home. We would be married three miles away, on Nauset Beach, on September 17, 2011. Robert and Irene planned a lobster bake under a tent the day before our reception. Both celebrations took place in our backyard. Finding a justice of the peace, scripting the ceremony, sending invitations and locating places for family and friends to stay, more than occupied our time and kept my focus away from my health.

Not What I Wanted to Hear

During a scheduled appointment at Sherry's office in Bridgeport, a few months before Mary and I were to be married, I was met with apprehension and surprise. "I think you're fine, but you should find out more about what's going on in your prostate." Sherry's words brought me to a place I didn't want to visit and was not embracing at all.

The urologist I spoke with at Mass General believed that what he felt during an exam was cancerous, that I should prepare myself and strongly consider surgery. Sam's urologist was more open to my views but was convinced I should choose between surgery or radiation, however, he would also consider watchful waiting.

Feeling uneasy after interviewing three urologists, I finally felt comfortable with a thoughtful, open-minded doctor at Yale. I became a patient of Dr. Thomas Martin that summer.

Did I ever want to have a urologist? No! It's curious how we view some things. "My urologist" infers he belongs to me; he is MY urologist. As much as I like and appreciate Dr. Martin, I would rather not spend time in his office. In my 40s, suggestions to see one after my third kidney stone attack, brought me to a chair facing the desk of a young doctor. As he talked, it didn't take long for him to lose me, particularly when he stated with utter conviction that he would be my doctor throughout my life. I had no intensions of adopting anyone, especially a urologist. I promptly left.

At the age of 61, with a life expectancy in the mid-80s, I learned that surgery wasn't the only option. Radiation treatments or watchful waiting should be considered as well. Each doctor suggested doing a biopsy. The mere thought of that sent shivers up my spine. My plan was to avoid this at all costs for as long as possible. Dr. Martin supported my desire to pursue alternative measures and to continue doing blood work. He never felt abnormalities during these exams. Apparently, the doctor at Mass General was wrong.

I would arrive for our consultations with apprehension surrounding my latest PSA numbers. Dr. Martin would soothe my nerves by sharing my score almost immediately. However, not wanting to heighten my mounting anxieties between appointments, I began to have the results of my blood work faxed to me. From the time I extended my arm, made a fist, watched the plastic band pulled tightly around my bicep and the vile of blood sealed and labeled, until my fax machine read "receiving" (three to five days later) more and more intrusive thoughts were laced with an unsettled, troubled imagination. Best case scenarios, relief or disappointment. *What do I need to do to get out of this situation? 62 is approaching.*

"When a PSA ranges from 0 to 4, there is no need to worry. If it moves above 4 we recommend a biopsy," Dr. Martin said during one of my appointments. I asked him to thoroughly explain what to expect during and after a biopsy, what the potential side effects were and if he had ever had one. I was looking for him to peel away what a trained doctor would say as well as not minimalize this procedure. Dr. Martin got my message. Even though he didn't have a firsthand experience, a more compassionate side revealed itself, which would serve us both well for a number of years. Attempting to convince myself that I was still okay, working toward acceptance that the biopsy would be negative, I agreed. Mary and I kept this to ourselves.

I AM TOO FAMILIAR WITH HOW YEARS CAN SEEM TO SLIP away and appear as though a single moment took its place. Time is merely a perception. It can stand still or be fleeting, move faster than we imagine. We sense it through a moving lens filled with our experiences. It can ground us as we tap into memories while attempting to hold on to what we cherish and allow us to dream as we glance at the future. I recall how I felt 22 years ago, using time as a buffer to detach from my father's journey. Now, here I am, almost there. What seemed like moments ago…

I began to spend even more time researching prostate cancer and what can be done to prevent it. But, I was hesitant to spend too much time because, by doing so, it felt like a concession, that I might have to admit I could become one of the 161,000 men each year who discover they have prostate cancer.

OUR CEREMONY

Two weeks after hurricane Irene made its way up the East Coast and swept through our yard, leaving behind a few downed locust trees, and power outages, Mary and I said our vows on Nauset Beach. A light breeze, cloudless sky and lowering sun accompanied seals as they swam not more than 30 feet offshore, peering above the waves like periscopes, watching our ceremony.

Forty friends and family members gathered on the beach while Mary and I posed for pictures in the parking lot as we waited for the signal to remove our shoes and stroll down the narrow boardwalk toward the water. We were to enter on opposite sides of our guests who were sitting on benches facing the water and the justice of the peace. We would walk past pots filled with tall feather reed grasses straddling purple lace hydrangeas, rose-colored lilies, wild irises and yellow sunflowers, and honor those loved ones who had passed; my mother, father and sister, Mary's mother, leaving flowers in the sand as we walked toward the justice of the peace.

Glistening, gentle ripples of water touched the shore, returning slowly back to a lazy tide. Distant squawks, the cawing of seagulls searching for remaining snacks or nodding their approval, left footprints that washed away with the next wave.

But wait!

Mary and I listened to loose planks creaking, watched four men in jackets and ties racing down the boardwalk, charging barefoot through the parking lot to a car. Evan was yelling, "Wardrobe malfunction! Wardrobe malfunction! We'll be right back."

Astounded at the site of Evan, Bryan, Robbie and a friend, it didn't take long for us to surmise that my plan had fallen through. In Bryan and Evan's haste to get to the beach on time, they must have forgotten. The day before, I had asked Evan to be my backup and to make sure Bryan brought the wedding bands to the ceremony. What was I thinking? Within minutes, the four slightly stressed, worse for wear amigos emerged from their car then ran back onto the beach and took their places in the sand. "You can start now," Bryan announced.

I faced my bride, taking her hands in mine, as the JP asked Mary to read her vows. I listened as Mary talked about a life together. "I will always be there for you." Resonating deeply, these words lingered so much so that I didn't hear most of what she said after that. I was touched, and never more convinced that my wife would walk by my side for the remainder of our lives. My emotions surfaced as I began to speak to Mary. I told her why I am so grateful we met, how much I loved her and how I looked forward to sharing our open hearts and dreams.

CELEBRATION AND A PROCEDURE

I couldn't believe we were doing this. Two weeks after our wedding, my PSA now above 4, Mary drove as Valium traveled through my bloodstream. I was in no condition to be behind the wheel. The closer we got to Dr. Martin's offices in New Haven, the less effective this dreamy drug seemed. The warmth of interlocking fingers as we walked to the office comforted me as much as knowing Mary was there.

I was awake and aware enough during the procedure to ask Dr. Martin for his opinion, based on what he saw. His response was promising and left me hoping that my 62nd year on this planet would not mirror my dad's. With post-biopsy instructions, precautions and a week of waiting ahead, Mary drove us back home.

By the time the Valium completely wore off, I was ambushed by lurking fears and doubts that intensified as the week progressed. Each day I questioned whether I should call Dr. Martin's office or wait for his office to reach out to me.

Should I aggressively pursue the results of this biopsy that could have a profound effect on my life? It wasn't a restful week and it was nearly impossible to mask my feelings or remain present, nor would it be the last time I'd be preoccupied with dying too soon.

"Some men choose not to know the results," Dr. Martin had shared during our previous consult. I began to appreciate this way of thinking. Once you get a cancer diagnosis, your life can change forever. You can't go back. My worst fears were influenced by the journey of my father and friends, as well as information I found on the web, often with intentions to alert the reader of the horrors associated with prostate cancer.

When my cell phone displayed a New Haven area code at 9:15 on Friday night, a week after the biopsy, my palms began to sweat, my eyes grew wider. Looking at Mary I said, "It's probably Dr. Martin." Tense and apprehensive, I answered.

Hearing Dr. Martin's calm voice helped somewhat. We both listened as he explained what was found. He began by saying, "While the lab did find something, the good news is that you will most likely die of something else, not prostate cancer." Hardly reassuring. Two out of 10 biopsied sections were inconclusive. There was no Gleason score. (A Gleason score measures the stage and aggressiveness of the cancer. The lower the individual number and the total, 3+3=6, is the most desirable.) A third section portrayed an early stage, non-aggressive form of cancer, a Gleason score of 3+4 = 7. The other seven sections were negative. Dr. Martin talked about probabilities, what a Gleason score means, options and suggested we schedule an in-person consultation.

Not too long after Dr. Martin shared the results, while still on the phone, I began to internalize, formulate and know with absolute certainty what I wanted to do. My reactions were instinctive and immediate. The times I'd spent in Sherry's office, and some of the research leading me to alternative views, brought me to the conclusion that cancer was an imbalance in my body. I believed that my body has an innate ability to reestablish that balance and would do so with proper support. Even though I was in a state of shock and enormously disappointed to be engaged in a conversation with a urologist about prostate cancer, I knew how I wanted to deal with this. To walk a different path, to find the answers I was searching for and to live a long and healthy life.

I did not acknowledge to myself or to Mary that I have prostate cancer. I was determined that the word cancer would not become part of my day-to-day vocabulary. Only Mary and I will know what led us to where we are, what we discovered and how this journey will unfold. I was adamant about this. "I do not want to be defined by cancer, viewed differently or randomly asked how I am feeling." As I spoke, I assured Mary that I was going to be okay and that we would have many good years together. With a fierce determination, emotions bottled up, holding back tears as anger surfaced, I took this information as a challenge.

Many factors affect the conclusion that the majority of men with prostate cancer will not succumb to this disease. Age at discovery, genetics, other health issues and treatments are all part of the equation. Before 2010, most men with a prostate cancer diagnosis elected to have surgery or undergo radiation treatment. There is evidence that their lives were extended, but how did the quality of their lives change?

While the news was relatively good, the far-reaching disappointment I felt knowing the biopsy indicated cancer was present, just as it had been with my dad, heightened my sensitivity to predisposition. I thought I had been doing all I could to prevent this and now I was overwhelmed by the need to dig in and fight. It's a challenge to be grateful when you and cancer are used in the same sentence. Instead of celebrating my apparent good fortune, namely that the cancer was non-aggressive, found early and relegated to a small area, my fight or flight reflex took over.

Yes, I did believe that I could realign my body, but I was reluctantly embarking on a new adventure and my doubts were deep-rooted.

<hr>

THE CONSULTATION

With a firm resolve to be my own best advocate and not to surrender to conventional medical options, I prepared for our follow-up appointment at Dr. Martin's office in November, two-and-a-half months after my 62nd birthday. Not knowing what to expect, I was determined to learn as much as I could before our consultation. My time on the Internet increased as I sorted through vast amounts of information, attempted to distinguish fact from promotions, scientific data from hearsay, promises from reality. I learned that prominent organizations and large companies can influence industries determined to help people with cancer by steering them in directions that lead to improved bottom lines and partial truths.

Even though Mary and I sat close to each other in separate

chairs, I felt isolated, but each time Mary said "we" as she asked a question or for clarification, my heart smiled, and I didn't feel quite so alone.

"There is a recent shift in the way we view treating men with early-stage prostate cancer," Dr. Martin explained. "We are not rushing to treat men surgically or with radiation. Watchful waiting, regularly scheduled exams, PSA blood tests are what we recommend. Considering how quickly the PSA number doubles is important to look at as well."

"What does that mean for us now?" Mary asked.

"You're okay," Dr. Martin assured us.

The energy in this small, sterile, sanitary room, its three chairs, exam table, sink and cabinets filled with supplies, changed each time Dr. Martin showed us his willingness to listen. He shared what he knew, answered all my questions, doing so with encouragement, helping us to digest the information as we sat through the two and a half-hour consultation.

Questions surrounding the PSA followed. How fast should the numbers rise? What numbers are considered safe after a positive biopsy? How often should I do blood work? I learned that the PSA blood test is not always reliable on its own, that there can be false positives. Horseback riding, bike riding and having sex within 72 hours of giving blood can cause the PSA to elevate, as well as other influences such as infections and even stress.

Dr. Martin explained all the current options and talked about potential new ways of addressing prostate cancer. These included technological and surgical advances such as high targeted radiation therapy and MRI-guided biopsies, as well as how rapidly new treatments were becoming available, and what the drug industry was doing to extend the lives of men with this diagnosis.

I was so far removed from considering any of this, except for watchful waiting. *Change the topic, move on.* As though a predator approached, my back rising, hair standing on end running the length of my spine, I was poised to challenge, or run.

"When do you believe we would have to think about this?" Mary asked. She was direct and relatively calm.

"You're okay for now, you're not in any danger," Dr. Martin stated assuredly.

He convincingly relayed that I should not worry and supported my efforts to actively seek alternative, nonconventional preventative avenues. We agreed that "watchful waiting" was my best option. Watchful waiting – poor choice of words – what was I watching and what was I waiting for? It occurred to me that I was waiting for the time to arrive when I would elect to be treated. My goal was to keep the quality of my life intact by avoiding traditional treatments, thus allowing my body to find the correct balance.

Driving in relative silence, we distanced ourselves from New Haven, stopping at G-Zen, a favorite vegan restaurant in Brantford. As we ate, Mary welcomed my thoughts. I continued to process our meeting and shared how I wanted to approach this challenge, attempting to be positive, all the while keeping my emotions in check.

"You know I support whatever you want to do." Kind words from Mary after a sip of organic wine.

"I appreciate that. I love you."

As we talked, I realized that I was attempting to convince myself as much as Mary that I would be fine, and I also knew this was the beginning of a potentially arduous road. There are many people who either give the impression or can actually compartmentalize their thoughts and feelings and make conscious decisions to live free of fear or concerns for their future. At this time, I can't say that I am one of them.

I MET THIS NEW LEG OF MY JOURNEY WITH HEIGHTENED curiosity, a sense of urgency and a desire to find potential causes and the most current traditional and nontraditional treatments. I examined the benefits of nutrition, diet, exercise, spirituality, bodywork and online support groups.

I broke things down into their simplest parts, identifying what efforts lead to success and removing extraneous information – becoming more efficient. This is how I ran my business. My attention to detail served me well in my quest to learn as much about prostate cancer as possible.

Almost robotic, with little creativity or joy, except when interacting with many of the librarians and media specialists who by now were friends, many workdays were not fulfilling or rewarding.

Finding a balance between running my business and gathering information became difficult. Full days of work could feel like a reprieve. I made a commitment to myself to keep informed and updated, but at times I was just tired of researching and felt conflicted. It became clear that surrendering to my waning passion for work was the answer.

Acknowledging this and the subsequent relief I felt proved invaluable and comforting.

SHORTLY AFTER RETURNING FROM OUR COSTA RICAN honeymoon in mid-February, we began to talk about selling the Old Lyme condo and moving into Mary's 1825 house on Cape Cod. This would mean relocating farther from our children, traditional doctors and the two naturopaths whom I now relied on to guide me.

When I began to seriously consider eliminating 30,000 miles of driving a year for face-to-face meetings, I was fraught with concern but at the same time excited. Would I be able to sustain my income level working remotely from Cape Cod? Giving up my condo and moving into Mary's home would also be a challenge. Her house was rich with family history — where she and her first husband spent summers, weekends and holidays together, raising their children. This charming place is similar to many homes in this town; weathered shingles, decades of coats of white paint, original doors and hinges leading from room to room in the midst of remodeled kitchens and bedrooms, wainscoting, hydrangeas and Cape roses. Cape Cod is magical.

What helped was Mary's willingness and encouragement, allowing me to see this 2-acre property as an easel to landscape, creating vegetable and flower gardens, opening dense tree-lined areas and replacing them with my imprint.

There was so much to do and so little time to worry. We continued discussing what could be done to make this home ours, and how I would take myself off the road, transitioning to working remotely. By early spring, we agreed that the benefits outweighed the risk and we put the condo on the market.

OUR PLANS WERE BRIEFLY INTERRUPTED A FEW MONTHS later when a simple cough exposing a small bulge above my groin diverted my attention long enough to interview two surgeons, weigh how I felt about them, and ponder what I had learned about hernia surgery. Often uncomfortable, at times in pain, I agreed that there were no alternatives. Early on a Tuesday morning, a few weeks into April, we found ourselves in New Haven preparing for hernia surgery.

It went well. A fairly quick recovery allowed me to pursue major landscaping projects and for us to oversee interior renovations with the hopes that most of this work would be completed by the time we moved in June. Everything we were doing, coupled with the good news that my PSA had gone down, provided a respite, temporarily freeing my mind from worry, allowing me to focus on our new life as husband and wife.

After living together for two years in the condo, we moved to the charming, sprawling Cape Cod home that has been in Mary's family for six generations. As I followed Mary in the rental truck filled with our lives, past and present, to our future in Orleans, I imagined this might be the last time I changed addresses. A pleasantly cool June day was met with some reservation, excitement and much anticipation.

SO OFTEN, THE VERY IDEA OF CHANGE CAN PARALYZE US,

fear of the unknown preventing personal growth. If we are able to move beyond this to that moment where we know that the risk or the fear is not the driving force, we can appreciate that the universe is in constant motion, changing and recreating all the time. Embracing this concept can be the impetus to move us to more readily welcome change. Easy for me to say when all seems right in my world and certainly a challenge to internalize when things are not.

I was spending less time educating myself about the latest prostate cancer research. With renewed passion, knowing I wouldn't be traveling for a living and that technology would steer my business, I vigorously planned the busy fall season. Delighted to find that all but a few media specialists and librarians agreed to continue working with me and help define my approach, I anticipated a successful transition.

As aging leaves revealed their bright fall colors, I still did not identify with cancer nor was I convinced that this disease was lurking within my prostate. Yet, I found myself back on the roller coaster. A rising PSA, close to 10, then down to 7.6 and back up to 11.4 exacerbated concern and anxiety. I visited Sherry more frequently. I also scheduled time in the office of Kendra, a naturopath steeped in science with fingertip information in Waterford, Connecticut. These appointments generated more remedies, supplements and advice from Sherry to look inside, to seek my spirituality.

I had learned from Dr. Martin that when a diagnosis of prostate cancer finds you, a PSA ranging from 4 to 10 is generally considered a safe zone, pending exams and reported symptoms. The absence of frequent urination or burning, few trips to the bathroom during sleeping hours, an ability to have erections and enjoy intercourse, all present as nonaggressive cancer, in most cases.

Prostate cancer is generally slow-growing and often non-aggressive. Depending on when it's discovered, many men can live productive, oftentimes symptom-free lives and never have to radically treat it. The tricky part is having enough evidence to make an informed decision about potential treatments.

"Tissue samples are our best indicator, follow-up biopsies, especially when a PSA rises steadily, is the procedure that provides the information we need," Dr. Martin said, attempting to gently persuade my thinking almost two years after I had my biopsy. "How long can you wait before you take steps to learn more than just what a PSA and exam might reveal?" Dr. Martin compared this to a game of Russian roulette. I didn't need analogies that fed my anxieties, but I completely understood. I was living this.

"A fluctuating PSA is not clear-cut evidence that the cancer has grown or become aggressive." Dividing men into two groups with divergent thoughts, Dr. Martin often talked about how men react to learning they have prostate cancer. "Let's aggressively treat this, get it out of me!" leading to surgery or radiation treatments. Or, "I want to postpone that decision for as long as possible." I was firmly entrenched in this latter way of thinking.

THINKING OBJECTIVELY HELPED ME FIND WAYS TO prevent cancer from spreading or deciding if I should aggressively treat it. Removing myself from the equation, which isn't always easy, helped me dispassionately review information with an open mind. At times, I felt forced to consider traditional treatments – and by doing so, hopefully extending my life. I would then be following my father's footprint more closely.

Toward the end, my dad had made his decision to forgo treatments that may have extended his life. The disease that continued to spread, his liver then affected, essentially removing hope, caused my dad to yield to the inevitable. I didn't want to find myself in the same position. It was so difficult for me to see beyond potential impotence, incontinence, emotional and psychological issues. Perhaps as important, I did not want to lose the ability to make love with my wife.

I still refused to acknowledge there was cancer in my body, even though my thoughts were not always cancer-free by now. And if there was cancer, there was no evidence it had spread. I had not been treated and my approach to life, diet, exercise and availing myself of alternative therapies all made my circumstances different than that of my dad's. Even so, I still believed I might have to choose between quality of life and life itself. This was primarily driven by PSA numbers and fear.

The times I shared these thoughts with Mary, I could see how burdensome and heartsick it left her. Because of my uncompromising decision not to share our discovery with anyone, not even our children, Mary often felt like she was on an island, isolated from friends and family who could offer a supportive ear, advice or a hug.

For this I am deeply sorry, Mary.

20

SOME LEARNING & A REPRIEVE

This part-time vegetarian was considering becoming a vegan. By now I was eating closer to the way I had wanted to for years. My research took me to vegetarian, vegan and juicing sites which led to finding the most reliable juicers on the market, specific recipes to attack cancer cells, and information about the best and worst environments for cancer. Abundant claims about juicing and its ability to cure a variety of cancers abound, so I bought a juicer.

I learned that cancer can't thrive in an alkaline environment. The more acidic our bodies are, the more opportunity for cancer to grow. Lemons, avocado, garlic, turmeric, broccoli and spinach can help maintain a balanced pH. Cancer also loves sugar, so it's important to eliminate sweets, even some fruits with naturally occurring sugars.

One of my major challenges, if I were to become a vegan, would be how to get enough protein. We already cooked with grains such as rice, quinoa and couscous, which do contain a fair amount of protein, but they can also be inflammatory. This can affect one's pH and contribute to other chronic diseases as well. Surprisingly, I discovered that many vegetables contain upwards of 2 grams of protein so juices, salads and cooked or raw vegetables can be valuable sources.

However, I felt a need to do more investigating before I made this commitment.

I WAS BECOMING IMPATIENT AND AGITATED AND IT WAS increasingly clear that Mary and I needed support. We often found ourselves at an impasse and weren't able to compromise or agree on a number of issues like what to have for dinner, when to spend time together, how often to have friends over or which movie to watch. Knowing I wasn't very accommodating, we found a couples therapist to help us navigate. We were back on strong footing after a few sessions.

A number of months earlier, as my personal journey seemed to be considerably impacting other parts of my life, I had begun talking with a different therapist. Feeling stuck as my PSA crept upward and my options appeared to be dwindling, I viewed these times to talk as a chance to say aloud what was bottled up. Even if the outcomes weren't going to change, at least I had a chance to express myself, perhaps gain new insights and share some of my deepest concerns.

AFTER A FOLLOW-UP APPOINTMENT WITH DR. MARTIN, I shared the results of the biopsy and what I had learned over the last two years with my closest friends, Steve and Meredith.

In some ways, I was bargaining with myself and inadvertently with Dr. Martin, Sherry, Kendra, Mary, Steve and Meredith. Searching for something promising that would boost my hope for a reprieve while postponing another biopsy, I looked for reactions and opinions and continued to accumulate data to make a strong case to stay on my desired path.

I discovered from the U.S. Department of Health and Human Services website that free radicals lead to cancer and that a variety of antioxidants (beta-carotene, lycopene, vitamin C, E, and D) can protect the body from damage caused by these unstable atoms. Armed with this information, I familiarized myself with foods high in antioxidants. Certain fruits (cantaloupe, papaya and pink grapefruit) and vegetables (sweet potatoes, spinach and kale), also some nuts, grains and even meats, fish and poultry are all great sources.

My research led me to the value of a pelvic MRI. This was another attempt to avert a second biopsy. "It's a way for us to collect more data, see where the cancer is and perhaps most importantly to use as a baseline to compare to subsequent MRIs, should we need them." Dr. Martin said. He responded to my request to do one after reviewing the history of my PSA scores, discussing new symptoms including occasionally getting up more often at night to urinate, but nothing else of any consequence.

Four and a half years into this journey, advocating for myself as much as my mother had for my sister, I scheduled a pelvic MRI in December of 2013 at Cape Cod Hospital. With a sense of relief knowing I'd avoided another biopsy, I was convinced proof that cancer didn't exist would appear on the images.

A well-trained radiologist can interpret the MRI, providing results at least as valuable as a biopsy. This was enough evidence for me. Because they don't section the entire prostate, biopsies can be inconclusive. This can lead to as high as 30 percent of men with no evidence of cancer, discovering later in life that they do, in fact, have prostate cancer. Potential side effects, such as bleeding, infection and the danger of moving cancer around, possibly spreading it, are real and don't apply to MRIs.

Attempting to drown out the loud noises, like jackhammers tearing apart city streets, and trying not to focus on urges to urinate, I lay on a cold, hard surface in an extremely tight-fitting tube, staying still for 45 minutes. Other than that, an MRI is not a bad experience. Especially compared to a biopsy.

HERE I GO AGAIN – LET'S START THE TIMER

Waiting for these results seemed different. I felt lighter and much more positive. My research led me to conclude that an MRI more firmly placed my destiny in my own hands. I was part of a smaller group of men participating in this fairly new approach, watchful waiting; not just waiting for something to happen, but actively uncovering unconventional means to address our body's imbalances. Because many men with prostate cancer will not die from it due to how slowly it grows, those choosing this path may continue to live as they always have.

. . .

WINTER CLOSED IN, BRINGING FADING LIGHT, FALLING temperatures, piercing winds and frozen ponds. Gray skies looked down on bulbs that lay dormant just inches below the frosty grass, biding their time, like sap sitting on a tree's base waiting to rise to the sweetness of spring. My spirits have dampened earlier and earlier over the years, as fall fades to winter, even more so as I navigated this journey.

Supportive as always, Mary agreed to spend some time in a warmer climate. A few weeks in the Caribbean one January, three weeks in Key Marathon the next, onto Key Largo after that. Not working much after 5pm these days, which three years ago had been inconceivable, I found my income remained essentially the same. Running my business remotely proved to be successful. More open to being away from my business allowed me to shift my belief that I had to endure long hours from September to July. I now felt I could step away, take a break from life's challenges.

A few days before leaving for turquoise waters and sunshine, the news came from Dr. Martin that the MRI was negative, confirming my convictions, stimulating my excitement, adding much relief. "This is good news. We now have a baseline. Let's follow up with bloodwork and an exam in six months," Dr. Martin said. Six months to live as carefree as I have in a long time, 180 days to change my lens and focus more on other things besides my health.

With each passing day I was less and less burdened. Lighter and happier. However, old habits can be hard to change. A pattern was established over four years – its seeds living in my past so gripping and ingrained – it was hard to let go.

. . .

AN OLD, COMFORTABLE, FADED BLUE EASY CHAIR SITS
between two windows, the wall displaying sketches of Bryan
and Evan as babies. My office faces the side yard and Mary's
Mother's Day crabapple tree, now 6 feet tall, and the berm
Steve and I designed, framing light green euonymus plantings
and a deep purple Japanese Maple. Family photos, books from
my past and those not yet read, a picture of Phineas, my first
golden retriever, and stacks of yearly tax returns are neatly
placed in the cabinet opposite my desk. Piles of catalogs,
sample books from my publishers, a fax machine and printer
all now sharing space, vying for my attention with an iPad,
often used to research prostate cancer. Random pieces of paper
noting what I'd recently discovered waited to be placed into
the file.

A new life had been created four years earlier, the day I
selected a plain off-white 8x11 file folder and began placing
copies of what I discovered while searching through the web.
Inanimate objects, mostly paper, came alive every time I
approached it. Thoughts intertwined with feelings, a relationship emerged. I had no idea how significant it would become.
Now, that file sat on the shelf behind me. Let it be. No need
to do blood work. Wait a while.

Anxieties heightened as time marched toward doing blood
work again. Approaching April, four months since the good
news, like an itch appearing out of nowhere, I reluctantly set
my sights on June, when I was to do blood work. I attempted
to ignore the urge to anticipate, trying hard not to buy into
old habits. Even so, there were many good days. New seeds to

sow, holiday celebrations, gardens to plan, golf and tennis to play. Dinners with friends and family, vacations to look forward to.

July neared and I wanted to stop thinking about my health. Summer's invitation, and my awareness that cancer was not found on the MRI allowed me at times to believe that I had nothing to be concerned about.

2 1

TELLING MY CHILDREN

When I said, "Come on over, I would like everyone to sit down at the table outside, there is something I want to talk about," eyebrows raised, smiles turned to serious faces, chatter to silence.

When we learned the results of the biopsy, my mission to prove that I can craft a happy ending began to take shape. I always believed if I was going to share my story, resulting smiles from those listening would accompany the ending. On occasions, Mary encouraged me to talk with our children. I was in a good place now and my reluctance faded. Feeling more confident and hopeful that my story would now have the desired outcome, I agreed to share our journey over a long July weekend in 2014 with Bryan and Evan. It happened that our friend Meredith was also visiting.

Room for us all, we eased into five wrought iron chairs surrounding a matching circular table. As we sat on our stone patio, I opened the umbrella to shade us from the midday sun. "What's up, Dad?" Evan anxiously asked.

Not everyone looked at me continuously, but they all listened intently as I filled them in, creating a chronology dating from insignificant, benign bloodwork, Sherry's guidance, to where I am now. I explained why I'd had a biopsy, the results, and the MRI, which was negative and looked toward Mary at times to add what I may have neglected to include.

"You know how much I trust her," I said, speaking to everyone, but in particular to Bryan and Evan. "During one of my appointments, a few years ago, as my PSA jumped, Sherry suggested I consider a biopsy."

When Evan asked what the number was, I took this opportunity to share what I had learned about this blood test and the fluctuations I've experienced. "The biopsy took place at Yale. It wasn't painful but the idea of it made me very uncomfortable."

The strained look on everyone's face matched my sentiments.

Charley, our 2-year-old golden retriever, snuggled up to Bryan. I couldn't be prouder of Bryan, and I'm not surprised that five years later, I would find him on the verge of becoming a doctor of psychology. His deliberate demeanor, thoughtful, supportive tones and caring personality will serve his patients well. Carefully choosing his words, my oldest son asked, "Do the results mean you have cancer? Are you going to be okay?"

"To me, it's inconclusive, but there was evidence. I firmly believe I'll be fine," I said without a hint of uncertainty.

Steeped in science, Evan relies on facts and numbers to

find answers to questions his curious mind seeks. A successful accountant by day, drummer by night, he moves to his own unique beat and often plays devil's advocate when my anomalous beliefs are the topic of discussion. My occasionally skeptical son, with his solemn look, didn't say much, but I could see and almost hear him processing all he had heard. "I know you believe in Sherry but are you sure you're doing the right thing?"

Looking in his direction, but telling everyone, I said, "Yes, I'm certain, Evan."

I paused from time to time to answer their questions and shared how strongly I believed this nonaggressive, early-stage cancer was an imbalance, and that I have been continuously working to aid my body, allowing it to make the appropriate corrections. "I don't identify as someone who has cancer."

This was a huge step for me. Talking about this openly with my children was so hard to envision. By doing so, I felt it legitimized the diagnosis three and a half years earlier. In responding as I did then, protective of my feelings, distancing from others, I took on this life challenge with a forceful energy and determination. Cancer would not be used in a sentence with my name.

I was finally sharing a secret Mary and I had held. Not disclosing what we knew had taken its toll. The burden of keeping something like this from my children removed, protective layers peeled away, I felt cleansed and renewed.

When Dr. Martin called with the biopsy results, I attempted to convince myself that I did not actually have cancer. A few years later, my thoughts would include, *If I do have cancer, I will keep it at bay.* And now, *Perhaps I didn't have cancer and maybe all that I have been doing has effectively removed any signs of prostate cancer from my body.*

Completing my story, I took this opportunity to educate Bryan and Evan with hopes that what they learned might serve them well if they faced similar decisions. I felt as good as I had in a number of years.

I was also pleased to keep my file out of sight on the shelf.

NOT WHAT I WANTED TO HEAR AGAIN

Having tripled in size, my garden demanded much attention and I was happy to spend my free time tending to it. A bountiful crop throughout the summer continued producing vegetables for our table late into the fall.

"We haven't had tomatoes this late in years," I offered, proudly carrying a Chestnut wicker basket to Mary as she stood in the kitchen preparing dinner.

"What else do we have?" Mary asked, smiling.

I unloaded my bounty onto the kitchen counter. "Japanese eggplant, pole beans, although not many – the rabbits got them first. Some carrots, and of course, lettuce."

I've grown lettuce for as long as I can remember and have enjoyed fresh salads from April to October. The rest of the year it hurts every time I open a plastic box of lettuce purchased from the supermarket.

We decided to greet 2015 in the warmth of Key

Marathon. Well aware that it had been more than six months since I stepped into Quest Diagnostics, I did so before we flew to Florida. Surprised to find my PSA was in the mid-teens, a jump of almost 4 points, I scheduled a phone consult with Dr. Martin. His composed reaction to my concern helped but couldn't alleviate the doubts that surfaced.

There were times during this journey, usually prompted by unwanted results, those damn PSA numbers, when I began to loosen my grip on what I strongly believed; that with help, my body would adapt and transform as needed, keeping me cancer-free. Like potential turning points, a road narrowing with no clear alternative path ahead, I felt as though unfavorable mounting evidence was too much to overcome. But, I always fought to remain positive. This was one of those times.

"If the MRI was negative, how could my PSA go up? What else could have affected the score? Do I have an infection?" Questions I asked myself and Dr. Martin.

"Let's do another PSA in a few months. It may be time to start thinking about other options," Dr. Martin responded.

Mary and I agreed to wait until we returned to the Cape in mid-February, hoping this was a temporary glitch.

Shortly after settling into the house we had rented, I decided to become a dedicated vegan. In addition to attending to my business, I spent a good deal of time reopening the file, revisiting what I had discovered and adding to the stacks of paper. I had hoped to never consult this file again.

I FELL OFF THE VEGAN WAGON A FEW TIMES AND consumed one last shrimp the day before we left Key

Marathon. When we arrived back down the Cape, my resolve to be a vegan was unwavering. Only organic foods, daily juicing, grains, sautéed vegetables, nuts, salads, no alcohol. Garden space would be taken up with kale, spinach, lettuce, beets, tomatoes, garlic, asparagus, beans and peas. I was determined to bring that PSA number down.

Mary supported my efforts, often sharing or discussing numerous interesting dishes for vegans. *I so appreciate your willingness to work beside me, thank you!* We ate this way for months as time continued to pass since my last results. If I were to do bloodwork, I expected a lower number. I was somewhat interested to find what that number would be, yet anxiety and fear prevented me from adhering to the timeline Dr. Martin and I had agreed upon. It was now 10 months since I last extended my arm.

Appointments followed with Sherry, Kendra and a new naturopath, Janet Beatty. Like layers of blankets keeping me warm on a winter's night, I believed another point of view and perhaps a different approach would comfort me. When I learned about Janet's bout with breast cancer, I felt connected to her in an unexpected way.

MID-NOVEMBER 2015

This fall, the sun seemed lower in the sky, earlier than usual. Once again, the onset of crisp, cooler air brought visions of the approaching winter and triggered my desire to escape. We planned our trip, but this time we would drive instead of fly. I would transport part of my office and actively set up space in the house we would rent for six weeks in Key Largo.

How many times in my life have I agreed to do something I was opposed to? Too many. Occasionally, it turned out to be in my best interest, other times, in retrospect, I'd realize that I had made the wrong decision. The higher PSA from last December was weighing heavily. Instead of doing blood work, I pushed for a follow-up MRI. "The equipment is more advanced at Yale than the machine used in Hyannis. Our MRI is more precise," Dr. Martin had explained. He convinced me to slide back into that tube the week before we drove south.

<hr>

JANUARY 2, 2016

Different circumstances revealed unexpected results. On the third day of our trip, near Miami, approaching the Keys as Mary drove, I spoke with Dr. Martin on the phone.

"It's difficult to know if what we found has changed in a year because the first MRI couldn't show what was discovered this time."

Mary listened intently while she drove.

"It's less than one centimeter. Not very big, but near the prostate wall." He went on to explain that with an elevated PSA and the current images we should have a conversation about treatment options. Dr. Martin assured me that I was not in imminent danger. "Enjoy your time in the Keys and schedule an appointment soon after you get back."

Reverting to a similar strategy, I bargained for more blood work with hopes of lower numbers and a potential follow-up

MRI. He agreed. Sobering as this was, my focus was on the small size of the tumor and the likelihood that prostate cancer is slow growing. Learning that it was close to the prostate wall was disconcerting. However, I recalled the results of the biopsy that suggested this cancer was nonaggressive and believed I was doing all I could to keep things in check.

Driving along this extended unique string of islands, we happily watched gulls fly overhead, pelicans glide inches from the water then dive beak first, capturing their lunch. We marveled as osprey tended to their young perched on man-made stanchions while gray and white herons plodded along shallow waters.

The Keys, stretching 120 miles from the southern tip of Florida between the Atlantic and Gulf of Mexico, surrounded by coral reefs and barriers, are phenomenal. Calm, warm waters display shades of turquoise, emerald and jade. Funky homes mirror ocean colors. Clusters of palm, magnolia and gumbo limbo trees cover the landscape. Our rental home safely tucked away from the ocean waters, its small private beach with canoe and kayak resting on a dock was visible from the living room and our bedroom. A pool awaited, steps away, protected by palm trees blending with exotic gardens, enhancing the beauty of this beach house.

"This is stunning," Mary said as she turned to see my expression.

I wholeheartedly agreed. "How fortunate are we?"

I practiced yoga every morning, breathing in the salt air, exhaling doubts. I walked or went to the gym each day, swam in our pool, read and napped on lounge chairs not far from the water's edge. My weekly hour-long drive to Whole Foods in Miami brought me in and out of civilization. On my way back, each time I crossed the bridge to Key Largo, my car brimming with bags of organic produce for our vegan meals and juices, I felt like I was entering paradise. It was easier to be present when each moment was surrounded by such beauty. It was a wonderful respite, yet I knew when we returned, I wasn't going to call Dr. Martin's office. My habits continued to be fueled by fear.

We returned to the Cape to a persistent cool, damp spring – yet again. I found myself fighting the elements while planting my garden, my passion for business diminishing even more so, working hard to stay in the moment but my efforts often thwarted. I was motivated to thoroughly enjoy the summer and had no desire to do bloodwork.

Even though I was looking forward to the array of visitors our home attracts each summer, many times I struggled to be fully present. When our last guests left in early September, as daylight began to dwindle, my ambivalence magnified. I was conflicted. Nagging thoughts crept into my vision laced with worry and concerns about decisions I didn't want to face, as well as the uncertainty of what this winter might bring. We delayed deciding where we would spend time when the cold arrived because I just didn't feel comfortable making a commitment, sensing I might have to do something I dreaded. Almost a year since my last bloodwork, I still haven't called Dr. Martin.

As I reached for the file, overflowing with information dating back to 2011, I lost focus. "There's so much stuff in here, look at all this!" I blurted toward an open window.

Suddenly, the file fell from my hand and dropped to the floor, scattering five years of research. Loose papers everywhere, printed information from the Internet sliding under my desk, newspaper articles and sticky notes lay scattered all around my office. "What the hell?" I screamed.

As my voice carried into the dining room and found Charley sleeping in his favorite spot, our faithful dog ran to my rescue.

"It's okay boy, I just need to be alone."

Charley left with his head down and tail between his legs. Hands covering my eyes, my head was already in my lap.

My anger thickened, congealing with frustration as I attempted to separate new information I had compiled this spring and fall from the mess on the floor; diets, blood and urine tests, wholistic retreats, and especially treatment options. I found myself moving from denial toward acceptance, continuing to be proactive.

I resumed my research. Risk versus reward was a significant issue for me. I talked with other men who had prostate cancer and began to interview doctors who had performed alternative procedures. Being appraised of potential short- and long-term side effects, their likelihood and severity was critically important and helpful.

I thought about surgery. But I immediately dismissed it. It didn't make sense at my age, now 67. Radiation therapy was the other standard treatment. Much to my disbelief, I left this door ajar. Additionally, within the relatively short time since I began educating myself, a number of advances in existing treatments had taken place.

Mid-October 2016

Another month had gone by, no bloodwork, no MRI, no discussions with Dr. Martin. Just research and anxiety. A foggy drizzle hovered outside as the embers in our wood-burning stove cried to be fed. As I added more wood, I turned to Mary, "I just don't want to make a decision that will compromise the quality of my life."

"I understand." Mary never questioned my desire to steadfastly walk the path I was on.

"I don't want to lose my ability to make love with you. I just don't want to be compromised." This was a huge issue for me. My unwavering manner, even as my PSA was rising, didn't outwardly appear to unsettle Mary.

"I love you." Words whispered in my ear as we embraced.

As delicious as this dinner has always been, on this evening, the vegetarian stew Mary prepared was difficult to enjoy.

There were times when I wish I had given Mary more opportunities to challenge my thinking. But I learned long ago, before we met, that my expressions, body language and certainty (not unlike my mother) can create obstacles for those attempting to get close to me. I set a tone, a semitransparent barrier. You're allowed to see just so much, get only this close, I won't show my vulnerability. But inside, I was aching to expose parts of me that lay dormant all these years, and to be open more often. It was important for me to feel in control, trusting I would make the right decisions. As I had before I shared my story with Bryan and Evan, I reverted back to old habits and kept from them what we learned in the past year.

23

I NEVER THOUGHT I WOULD
BE HERE

The shadows of potentially choosing life or death shrouded the room. The gravity of this somber meeting lingered like mist falling through gray clouds, penetrating my thoughts. When it was over, I was even more determined to find an acceptable treatment.

I'm not sure why I agreed to put myself through this. Maybe out of respect for my therapist's views and perhaps, more importantly, for confirmation. Barbara, also trained as a nurse, suggested during one of our sessions, "Why don't you consider meeting with an oncologist, just to gather more information?"

I took her advice and scheduled an appointment with a radiation oncologist, three months after my 67th birthday.

"Oncologist," hearing or repeating that word fueled the beliefs I was so deeply holding onto and my concerns about traditional medicine's approach. In my heart and soul, I knew I wouldn't seriously consider radiation, but I agreed to go.

Holding Mary's hand, I hesitantly walked into Cape Cod Hospital. I didn't want to be here. Not unlike I had felt entering the armory, 37 years earlier. We listened as a well-spoken, educated, convincing middle-age doctor spent two hours in an office equipped with props, chalkboard and slides, presenting as a lecturer what his beliefs were as Mary and I attempted to take it all in.

I know his intentions were good and it was clear to me that the potential outcomes he presented, if I did nothing, were meant to scare as much as inform us, perhaps into making hasty decisions. "There is little possibility that you will live a long, productive life if you don't treat the cancer," our presenter stated. He continued our education with comparisons to various treatments, surgery and seed implantation among others, always coming back to the advantage of a five-day a week, four-month course of radiation.

We left frightened, confused, but better informed. I was even more convinced that radiation wasn't for me and I hoped with every living, thriving cell in my body that I wouldn't be forced to seriously consider it.

"Why don't we think about going to Naples, Florida, this winter?" I asked Mary during a quiet dinner this late autumn.

JANUARY 3, 2017

The PSA went up again, now in the low 20s.

Bad news, like winter, is something I can do without. A week before we left for Naples, the results of another MRI at Yale, using the same equipment as the previous one, revealed the tumor was now closer to the prostate wall.

"I think it's time to make a decision." These words spoken by Dr. Martin just days before we finished packing stopped me in my tracks.

Five years earlier, when the word cancer had been used in the same sentence as my name, my conviction and certainty had guided me. As hope splintered and my options appeared scarcer, my despair heightened.

The enthusiasm attached to a pending respite from the cold was extremely difficult to find. Once again I consulted the file, searching for rays of light, this time focusing primarily on treatment options both here and outside of the country.

The file in my backpack accompanied me on our flight to Florida. I had every intention of not letting it out of my sight. Boxes filled with what was needed to run my business arrived a few days after we pulled into the driveway of our rental home. Lacking enthusiasm, I walked through the motions of setting up my office.

I began sharing some of my thoughts and feelings with Dr. Martin. Over the next several weeks we continued to exchange emails and talk. I closed an email in January stating that, "I believe my best option to address my prostate cancer is high intensity focused ultrasound or focal laser ablation therapy. I am grateful for your support. Thank you, Dr. Martin." Both procedures use a source of energy: heat, cold or lasers, to kill cancer cells.

Sitting at a glass table in a small screened-in porch, I contemplated what I knew to this point, while geckos defied gravity as they climbed, darted and stared from their mesh perches. By the middle of January, I believed I was ready to make an informed decision.

Information about alternative clinical trials came across my screen, most of which combined some form of traditional treatment such as radiation therapy. Because research is ongoing, new discoveries, therapies and procedures will undoubtedly expand – but *my* time was running out.

I also considered checking into a healing center such as the Hippocrates Health Institute, in West Palm Beach, where they believe, as Dr. Atul Gawande wrote in "Being Mortal: Medicine and What Matters in the End," that disease is a mere snapshot of one's current state caused by epigenetics (lifestyle).

JANET BEATY'S JOURNEY COMES TO AN END

In mid-January, while in Naples, the news from Janet Beaty took me by surprise and heightened what I was feeling about my own journey.

"I trust and believe in my oncologists. My choices were limited, and the treatments were difficult to tolerate." This was just some of what Janet shared with me while talking on the phone about chemotherapy and other approaches to treat her cancer last winter.

I would learn from Janet that her "spring cleanup," as she termed it, an effort to eliminate as much as possible of the cancer that remained and was still compromising her health, had brought her close to death. "I was this close to dying!" I imagined the space between Janet's thumb and pointer finger narrowing as she spoke.

The reality of her struggles with cancer now so clear to me, further enhanced my sensitivities to standard treatments and demonstrated on such a deep level how horrifying this disease can be, often leading to decisions we would never want to consider. In an effort to offer support and hope, I shared some of my discoveries, particularly what I'd learned about healing retreats.

I flashed back to how I felt a few years before, when we had reconnected, and I'd first learned that Janet had breast cancer. *How can someone who views medicine through a shifting lens, open to and treating her patients with alternative means, who's so knowledgeable about herbs, remedies, supplements and creates such beauty in her flower gardens…ever get cancer?* The irony.

It's unjust and unfair to find a healer stricken by cancer. Fundamentally, it didn't make sense. Unrealistic? Yes. Child-like? Perhaps. But a thought nonetheless that occurred to me, bringing me closer to Janet and frightening me even more.

The summer of this year would find Mary and I attending a memorial gathering at Janet's home with friends and family members celebrating her dedication, compassion for her patients, fondness for animals, and her joy of life. The outpouring of love, affection and admiration was heart-warming and wonderful to be a part of.

Gone too soon.

24

ANOTHER SOBERING APPOINTMENT

January 23, 2017. In the midst of my adversity I reached for rays of light, while grasping onto hope. Every time my PSA unexpectedly rose, or an MRI revealed an enlarging tumor, I latched onto anything positive. I expected good news from Dr. Sperling.

A few weeks after arriving in Naples, I decided it was in my best interest to visit the Sperling Center in Delray Beach to discuss Focal Laser Ablation Therapy. We embarked on a two-hour drive across Alligator Alley. A numbing sensation prevented me from being completely present.

With overtones of 47 years ago when I considered joining the Army Reserve, and memories from this past November, hearing but not digesting what the oncologist presented, we found ourselves in a cramped medical office. Dr. Dan Sperling explained the procedure and began to view my MRI, now clipped to a screen on the wall. The conversation took on a more somber note as he explained how close the tumor was to the prostate wall and how he in fact suspected that cancer was outside the wall and elsewhere in my body. My heart dropped.

I was sitting in a chair facing the doctor I thought would offer me the best chance to eradicate what was growing in my prostate, using a relatively noninvasive procedure without radiation. Now, doubt surfaced that I may actually be a candidate. The consultation moved to alternative treatments, one of which took place in Holland, as well as a five-day course of radiation. Fortunately, Dr. Sperling agreed that he could help. There was a slot open for the procedure in early February. We took it.

The ride back to the house was all too familiar. We talked about Dr. Sperling's suggestion that I do a bone scan, which was part of the protocol to rule out if cancer had spread. I wasn't in favor of doing this due to the amount of radiation exposure and what it might reveal. We also discussed if I would consider radiation therapy.

Forlorn, dispirited and beyond disappointment, I turned to Mary as she drove. "I don't know what to say. I didn't expect to hear this."

"Neither did I. Dr. Sperling did say he could help. I know you don't want to do a bone scan. Will you do it?"

Having this new information and feeling somewhat detached, I found myself considering this. Choosing between life and death suddenly became more real. I talked with Mary about the pros and cons of ablation therapy, other alternatives, and if I would actually keep the appointment and have the procedure. Even in the face of what we had just learned, it was so hard to break old habits. All that I read about ablation therapy took on life now. The more we drove, the further I distanced myself from the idea of doing this. *How can I get out of it? What else is there? Can I wait until research meets my needs and desires? Find the file when we get back!*

AN OPPORTUNITY TO GUIDE SOMEONE ELSE - A GIFT

My son Evan had introduced me to Melissa three weeks before we left for Naples. Her husband Joe, and Evan are band mates and good friends. I needed someone to help move boxes of books into a number of libraries and with two young children and the holidays approaching, Melissa and her husband, could use some extra money.

"Tell me more about your business." Following up with Melissa, we talked a few days after Mary and I had met with Dr. Sperling. Melissa was curious to know more than I had shared with her in December, and I was happy to paint a picture of my life as an educational consultant. A frank, honest, open discussion laid the framework for our relationship. With options dwindling, discouraged and downhearted, my spirits lifted each time we talked. It would be four months until we spoke again when I would learn that Melissa was seriously considering working with me and eventually running my business.

Speaking with God, so vulnerable, looking for a miracle, I felt as though something had died within me when my prayers weren't answered – too young. At 7, I began an oftentimes lonely journey, navigating through my insecurities, molding my masks, and creating a persona that best suited my needs. I lost faith and began stepping away from my sister. However the relationship I had given up on, still had much to teach me.

How Mom must have felt in that moment when she resigned herself to a fate similar to that of her mother's. Lingering in her subconscious; a reminder of what she thought awaited her at age 56 – too soon. *Disregarding your health, living as you wanted, counting the years, but thankfully finding a grander purpose shortly after your daughter was born. Devoting your life from 35 until your passing at 85 and beyond to teaching Ronda and others about life. Heartaches and victories, blazing trails with and for other parents; teaching, always teaching.*

The fright in that moment, gun to your head, not knowing if what you say or do activates an impulse and causes the man holding you up to squeeze the trigger out of fear or rage. Did you think this was too soon Dad? I imagine you thought you weren't ready any number of times as you lay in a hospital bed, or minutes removed from a doctor's consultation, in quiet moments wondering, reflecting – too soon?

And when, in your 73rd year, on the last walk you and Mom would take from a doctor's office, did you begin to accept that your time was nearing? Did you anticipate what lay before you as desires and joys began to fade? Did you agree it was time? Were you afraid of dying? Did you arrive at a peaceful place?

When entering the Armory's hallway as a 20-year-old, my

imagination had opened to damp heat and rice fields surrounded by mud. I could see myself in those newspaper articles and television reports from the battlefields in Vietnam. So disturbing, these unsettling images scared this young man, bringing me closer to facing death – too soon.

Mom, a few weeks before you left this earth, I was taken away while sleeping, the dream so real and confirming what I believe – that there is much more beyond this life. I was brought from my house, transported through time and space within a blinding light back to my kitchen, surrounded by deceased family members. Peaceful souls sitting and waiting. Your father stout, so tall, looking over everyone, all in what appeared as a fog while they anticipated your arrival.

A week before you passed on, those whispered words, "I don't want to go," left me questioning what you really meant. After all you had been through, nurses, doctors and me believing the battle would soon end, did you think it was too soon? Were you afraid to leave, moving on to a new reality?

The day after arriving home from our last visit, I stood in my shower. You appeared. Mom, seeing you again, your wanting eyes looking back at me seemed to ask if it was your time. "It's okay to go Mom, you can let go," I whispered with my eyes closed. A few days later, we both knew you were ready.

Ronda, I hope it wasn't too soon. How painful it is to imagine what you went through the day the sixth message on my machine beckoned me to look deep within. I searched for guidance and attempted to make sense of what happened to you, just weeks before your 55th birthday. I want to believe this was a peaceful passing. That it was indeed your time and the work you came to do was completed, and that on some level, you knew that and took solace in your journey's end. I hope so.

Mary's Thoughts Imagined

I often worried what Mary was thinking. *Responsibilities taken on lovingly. But nonetheless a growing burden. Moving through guilt and resentment. Confusion stopping me in my tracks. I wonder how we got to this place. How do I stay connected with an open heart and tethered soul as your body fades? I miss us. This is so hard…the man I love and married only a handful of years ago followed the path he believed was best for him. I do respect your decisions. But what about me…what about us? Why didn't you do something sooner? Yes, your lifestyle may have been compromised, as well as ours. But, I want more time together.*

My Thoughts

Sheer terror penetrated through every cell in my body as I envisioned awaiting the results of the bone scan. Visualizing what my life would be like if cancer was found gnawing on these bones. Imagining, in the minutes before Dr. Sperling called back, the effects chemotherapy would have on my tissues, organs, psyche, not to mention what was left of my lifestyle. These visions so real, so powerful, my body shaking, cold sweat turned to heat then back to cold again. "Please let the phone ring, I can't take it anymore!"

Within those moments, death staring me right between

the eyes, calling me much too soon, I didn't feel ready to leave this life behind. My most deep-rooted fear was dying now, when it wasn't my time yet, not the fact that I was going to die, although I wasn't exactly excited about that idea either. I wasn't ready to say goodbye to Mary, friends, my children or to anything that stirred an emotion, touched my heart, and confirmed my humanness. So deeply saddened, I was horrified that I found myself enmeshed in these thoughts.

Do we all get a glimpse at the approaching transition when we realize there is no turning back? Whether someone is taken too soon, too quickly, or if we live a full life with time to reflect. The vision is so clear. Just as I was about to submit, turning my control over to the inevitable when I walked into that dark room, I lay face down on the MRI table and waited for the ablation procedure to begin. I was between two worlds, placing my trust in a doctor and his staff, equipment and a procedure that would hopefully be transformative.

When we die, the body decays, like leaves in autumn falling to the ground. Life-sustaining energy gone as we pass on, facing the unknown, carried along and transformed into a different existence. Perhaps the soul's purpose is to guide us with intentions of welcoming us back, as we shed our earthly experiences and continue to move closer to God. And the cycle continues moving back to when a speck removed becomes a spark of new life.

For a long time, I believed the soul existed somewhere within the universe. I now imagine it exists within all dimensions, evolving within us while we're on earth, taking the good that serves its growth, brightening as it fills with kindness, compassion and love.

And I know, when I die, that I would like to feel complete. Regrets long gone, purposeful days that followed, my most recent memories satisfying, content and peaceful, surrounded by love.

2 5

MORE GIFTS

I believe with absolute certainty there are no coincidences. If I remain open and look carefully, my intuition can expose pathways leading to guidance.

Days before the scheduled ablation therapy I remained uncertain. So what else is new? I continued to grasp for other solutions and was curious about the Omni Center, a spa offering alternative mind/body therapies. I was grateful when I arrived that the owner suggested I meet with Dawn, a spiritual healer, rather than avail myself of the many other services they offered. As I sat in Dawn's office, I learned of her near-death experience as a young woman and her subsequent calling to help others. I shared my journey with Dawn and energies were set in motion that had a profound effect on both me and Mary.

More than one miracle changed everything. Hesitant but agreeing to do a bone scan, I battled to make a case to myself that the risk of radiation was outweighed by the information it would provide. "Do you have any metal in your body? A belt, credit cards, ammunition or guns? If so, please place them on the chair," the technician instructed.

Anticipation was replaced by some relief when I walked out of the diagnostic center. "Look for the results in two to three days. Your doctor will contact you," the assistant announced as I was leaving.

As soon as I began my drive back to our rental home, relief quickly morphed back into worry. There was a lot more at stake. I was not prepared to conceive of the possibility that a relatively small amount of cancer in my prostate, slowly growing, would ever move from this gland.

The phone rang later that afternoon.

"The results of your bone scan are here. Dr. Sperling will call you back in a few minutes to discuss them," the administrator at Dr. Sperling's office said.

You have got to be kidding me! Can't you put him on the phone? Why not tell me what it shows? I was stunned by the call, two days before it was expected, and terrified to know the results.

I felt frozen in space. Horror kept my heightened anxiety company. My mind raced. *Why didn't she just tell me they didn't find anything? Maybe she's not legally allowed to disclose the results? It must be bad news, why else would she call and not put the doctor on?* Only Mary can describe my ashen color, lifeless appearance, empty stares, disconsolate energy.

I have buried the next 20 minutes of my life before Dr. Sperling called back so deep within my soul that it would take a miracle to unearth it.

When my cell phone rang again, showing the same

number it had before, the cliff I stood on trembled. Through the speaker, Mary and I heard Dr. Sperling happily report the results of the bone scan were negative. He went on to say that he now believes ablation therapy will eradicate the prostate cancer and that there probably isn't cancer anywhere else. Two miracles.

I could feel the warmth of the day once again, and the possibility that this reluctant journey would soon end. But not quite as I envisioned.

Mary was preoccupied, not just due to what we were facing at this time, but because of pressures at work, and it was increasingly difficult for me to be there for her. Later that day, Mary found me in another part of the house. She approached me overjoyed, grateful and absolutely delighted to inform me that a huge obstacle at work cleared a path for her to move ahead on a project she wanted. We both felt lighter for the first time in a while.

I don't believe we intentionally worry our children. I believe as they grow along with us, we as their parents continue learning how to support, teach and guide them, always being there. It wasn't my mother's desire to put me on alert, subconsciously watching and waiting for her 56th year to arrive. Nor did my father plan to discover he had cancer at 62, knowing his son would internalize this, setting his sights 28 years into the future.

Maybe all of us know on some level what we came here to do. Perhaps we just can't remember how we agreed to help others as well as who is here to show us what we need to learn and what surprises, hardships and special moments will be the trigger to free our souls. For many of us, accepting that life can be difficult at times is part of the learning. Most of us don't get a free ride, except maybe the few evolved souls, back for one more stroll.

———

FEBRUARY 4, 2017

My dad's first cancer treatment was at 62. Now 67, Mary and I stepped into Dr. Sperling's office and waited. Brief moments of wishing this away followed. I so desired to leave this waiting room and push open the glass doors leading to the fresh air outside. Random thoughts appeared out of nowhere and just as quickly evaporated, making room for the next one. Attempting to make sense of everything, I was assessing my life as it seemed to flash before me.

"Where are you? What are you thinking?" Mary asked as she placed her arm in mine.

"Why is it taking so long? Let's get this over with," I said. Mary moved closer.

My journey had brought me here. To a small imaging center on the east coast of Florida. To a shared waiting area that opened to a dark bare room where the procedure would be performed. We had agreed with Dr. Sperling that he would do a biopsy immediately after I was prepped. It was important to get a Gleason score before the ablation procedure eradicated the cancer.

Even though friends and family had offered advice,

encouragement and support, bridging the gap of time between thoughts, sending me their love – as this journey neared an end, I felt stranded. Alone on a remote island surrounded by water, watching particles of sand, like moments in time, erode, slowly disappearing as the ocean advanced. All the while knowing the tide would not retreat – and I didn't know how to swim.

Yes, I agreed to have the procedure, but I was still fundamentally against admitting that cancer resided in my prostate. I didn't want to treat what was revealed on that last MRI any differently than I had so far. My insides were kicking and screaming, like voluntarily entering a nightmare but hoping to wake up before it begins.

The Valium only temporarily masked what I believed; that I had let myself down. I was responsible for not finding the answers. Is this feeling so deeply rooted? Similar to how I felt when I believed God let me down?

If Ronda were here, she would say, "I love you." That simple. I now know it would have been her way of saying, "You didn't know that you weren't supposed to change me. You were to learn how to love me, embrace me for who I was. But you couldn't have known that when we were so young. Everything was so fresh, so new. Yes, that did change, and challenges were in front of us. That's the way it is. Life is about learning to love. I have long since forgiven you and have always loved you. Thank you for being there when I needed you most."

I am finally at peace with this.

A few years after Ronda came into the world, I ran from her and pursued a confusing journey that took me away from my true self. For the past six years I have run toward knowledge, looking for answers, finding my way back. Can I finally forgive everyone I blamed…most importantly me? Will I then be able to return to my authentic self?

When we were called in, Valium working overtime to temper my nerves, the procedure and recovery explained, I finally yielded. There was no turning back.

1:30 A.M.

"Hi honey, how are you?" Mary asked, smiling.

She was sitting next to a nurse in the same cramped, cold room where I had removed my clothes and handed over my cell phone in what seemed like an eternity ago. A few minutes later, I felt as though I was going to pass out.

An hour later, Dr. Sperling came into our room and reported that the procedure was successful.

Mary and I finally walked out those glass doors to a surprisingly cool night and drove to a nearby hotel so I could recover for a few days. Upon returning to Naples, I heeded advice to refrain from working out and lifting more than 20 pounds for a while. I allowed my body to heal, gradually introducing yoga and short walks. I practiced patience when progress took a momentary step back. For weeks afterwards the relief was palpable. The procedure and everything it represented was behind me.

My research paused when I discovered ablation therapy.

But, if I was to have the procedure I knew it wasn't all I would do. Once I took my first running steps that day at the Bronxville track, my focus changed. All these years, the supplements, remedies and advice had a cumulative effect on my thinking and beliefs, and there still was more to learn. Since ablation therapy removed the cancer, I now had an opportunity to start fresh and an obligation to do all I could to give this body the best chance to thrive.

Late February, not quite a month after the procedure, still in Florida, tired and happy to read or just sit outside, I meditated on the porch. I believed it would be a challenge to go out with Mary and our friends, yet I reluctantly agreed. When we arrived at the restaurant, to my surprise, I was happy to share a meal with Lorrie, Mark and Mary, and felt grateful for the time together.

A number of months had passed since I spoke with Sherry or Kendra. Mark introduced me to a homeopath named Kent. Forthright, inquisitive and soft-spoken, Kent asked me questions geared toward understanding who I am on many levels. Health histories, life's traumas, food preferences, allergies, experiences, how I react in certain situations and more. All in an effort to find the correct remedy to address my desire to eliminate cancer from my vocabulary, and to maintain a healthy balance. I was pleased to hear about a remedy called thuja, just one teaspoon a day, and found Kent's recommendation and generosity in spirit and time comforting.

By the late spring, I still felt there was more to learn, perhaps because it was difficult to trust a single dose of this remedy would have the ability to do so much. I asked Kent about functional medicine – another alternative practice. He was more than willing to share what he knew. I began to research this approach, leading to several doctors in Massachusetts and a conversation with Kent's recommended practitioner in New Jersey.

Temperatures were in the low 80s when we left Naples mid-March, a month and a half after my procedure. We returned to the Cape, temperatures in the 40s, overcast skies and another spring not yet ready to bloom. This was to be my last busy work season. I went through the motions, scheduled fewer appointments than usual, while still recovering, and began to envision life outside and removed from 17 years as an educational consultant. I also relished the idea of mentoring Melissa. Much planning, trainings, meetings and conversations with clients prepared everyone for the transition.

THREE MONTHS AFTER THE PROCEDURE, AS MY BURDEN of concern eroded, I scheduled my follow-up appointment at Dr. Sperling's office for bloodwork and an MRI. Mary and I also began seriously considering buying a house in Naples, Florida. One of Mary's gifts is her willingness to remain open to my ideas. This was a big one! Knowing how I had grown tired of winter, its stunted days and frigid air, Mary entertained my latest brainchild, which helped to positively reframe this part of our journey. I was glad to find something exciting to focus on that brightened a memory and diverted my attention.

Each morning at our hotel, I woke at 4 a.m. I felt called to meditate and found when I opened my eyes there was a clarity that soothed and guided me. We spent two days looking at houses with our realtor, the third at Dr. Sperling's office. The PSA went from 26 to 17, the MRI showed no signs of cancer. I felt as positive, confident and as calm as I had in a long time. Yet, I knew doubts still lurked.

It is virtually impossible to change some things, let alone modify what feels like inherent behaviors. "How fast should the PSA go down and what number would convince us that there is no cancer in this body?" I asked.

"I would like to see it below 4 and it can take up to a year," Dr. Sperling replied.

Why was I at 17? For comfort, I relied on what we just learned. The MRI was negative and the results of the biopsy performed immediately before the ablation procedure, disclosed a Gleason score of 3+3 equaling 6. This also cast a shred of doubt and reminded me I had never been completely convinced that cancer was even present. How can my Gleason score go from 3+4 to 3+3? Yes, cancer may have been present, but was it possible that this slowly growing tumor was losing its strength?

I WANTED TO MOVE THROUGH TIME, BACK TO THE moment before my cell phone rang that Friday evening on the Cape or to the second before I gave blood for my physical eight years ago. To just before I learned of the melanoma behind my father's right eye. To the afternoon we stood at my grandmother's grave site, my mother about to share her concerns. To the minute before I listened to the voice of

Ronda's caregiver on my answering machine 14 years ago. To joyous times of celebration when my children were born. Back to summery Sundays at Bay 35 in Coney Island. To any time in my life when a given moment's boundaries are removed, leading only to the next moment.

I knew I couldn't turn back time. But how do I learn to live with my past, to embrace my journey, continuing to acknowledge each lesson and move beyond the fear, finding a place of comfort where I can rest in the pure light of that moment? If cancer brings me there, then all I have been through has been worth it.

CAN DOUBT LEAD TO AN UNDESIRED OUTCOME?

October of 2017, Mary and I sat in our backyard on Cape Cod gazing at the sky. That night, hurricane Irma was to make landfall on Fort Myers Beach, where we had bought a home a mere four months before. Almost simultaneously Mary saw a shooting star as I viewed another one racing across the sky in a different direction.

"Did you see that? I just saw a shooting star!" Mary shouted as I echoed her words.

That's when we knew our house would be spared the devastating, widespread destruction reported in so many parts of Florida over the coming days and weeks. Feeling extremely grateful and blessed, we appreciated how fortunate we were. And once again, I felt there was more to life than what exists here on earth.

"There are three things you want to refrain from doing at least 72 hours before you give blood that can affect the PSA; biking, horseback riding or sex." Dr. Martin's words. According to Dr. Sperling's guidelines, I was due for blood-work three months after the last tests. I would like to say I had no reservations or doubts. I believed the number would go down but also wondered if it would be low enough to satisfy me.

I left Quest Diagnostics with a fresh bandage on my left arm shortly after 7 a.m. on Saturday morning. Two days later, Dr. Sperling's office called and reported that the PSA had gone up to 22.4.

How could that be? Stunned by the news, disappointed and dismayed, I asked Mary to call Dr. Sperling's office. When the nurse picked up, Mary handed me the phone, "It's not uncommon. Any number of factors could contribute. Do it again in a month," she said. Working through my confusion, Mary and I began to talk. She confirmed what I believed, that we had made love the Friday night before I gave blood. "I'll take that explanation," I said with a large grin on my face.

Even so, I wasn't 100 percent convinced this was the reason and it would be more than a month before I gave blood again. Searching for other explanations, I decided to more intensely pursue additional support. My journey was moving in a new direction and the universe was getting my attention, guiding me to veer from the path I was traveling.

The news this fall that my PSA stood at 22.4 delivered a message and propelled me to look more carefully at functional medicine. My research led me to Dr. Linda Reynolds, who integrates Eastern, Western and European health modalities. She also incorporates the art of Ayurvedic, a traditional system of medicine originating in India, and quantum healing, which combines principles of mind-body medicine with ideas from quantum physics.

For so many years, even though my beliefs led to alternative practitioners, my mindset was more traditionally based, trained to think a certain way. Western medicine treats symptoms, not the cause and doesn't consider the whole person. Mucinex for clogged sinuses, aspirin for a headache, Pepto-Bismol for an upset stomach, an antibiotic for an infection. The pharmaceutical industry has created thousands of medications to address symptoms but bypasses the causes.

For years, sitting with bloodwork, looking for imbalances, discussing my concerns and desires, Sherry, Kendra and Janet had suggested a variety of remedies to help rebalance my body. These well-intentioned, incredibly smart women took a different approach. I learned so much and am extremely grateful they have been such an important part of my life. But it's clear to me that traditional medicine's approach affected my thinking. Placing a supplement or homeopathic remedy under my tongue or in my mouth, much like an aspirin or antibiotic, was the answer. I relied on these natural remedies and believed my body would find its own innate ability to heal itself. However, I wasn't fully embracing the entire picture – the whole me.

My faith in nontraditional therapies and my beliefs were so strong, it may have bought me time. However, my desired results before the procedure, ridding myself of any signs of prostate cancer apparently weren't coming to fruition. The nagging uncertainty, discontentment and longing to make sure I was well informed so that I could make correct choices lingered – always looking for answers. Something was missing.

By no means am I an authority on the subject of cancer. I witnessed my father's journey with this disease, as a melanoma discovered behind one eye relied upon the unfortunate wisdom that is characteristic of cancer – its ability to stimulate its own growth and spread years later. Cancer cells are essentially immortal. In addition to my research, I have read about celebrities', athletes' and other people's battles, talked with several friends and learned of their families' struggles with cancer.

Cancer has lived through the generations, described by the Greek physician Hippocrates in 370 BC and found in mummies in ancient Egypt as far back as 1600 BC. I don't know if there is a more comprehensive plan for all of us. Everyone at some point is touched by cancer – a family member, friend, coworker, mother, a child, someone we meet on a street corner. Are we here to learn something from this insidious disease?

What do we suppose are the lessons? I believe, as biologist and author Bruce Lipton does, that "biochemical effects of the brain's functioning show that all cells of our bodies are affected by our thoughts. That by changing the environment, namely our thoughts you can change the activity of cells...even cancer."

So, is it possible that three or four years ago, when concern, doubt and fear fought for and eventually occupied more of my thoughts, converting my convictions and strong beliefs, that I then began to lose the battle? Is that when my environment changed enough to allow this awful disease to gain momentum? Is this the answer, or part of it?

Will learning how to better care for our planet, becoming advocates for climate change, removing harmful chemicals and toxins essentially found everywhere from the soil to the beds we sleep on each night be helpful? I believe so. Should we listen to alternative views, even if it means huge industries with more concern for their bottom lines than our well-being will lose their control and power? Most definitely!

The environment outside ourselves includes the food we eat, planted and harvested from the soil on farms around the world. The air we breathe, everything we see and hear. What our taste buds tell us and everything we touch. We can choose complacency or action – and change if we so desire it.

We can buy organic food, purify the air in our homes, clean up the air in our cities or live in the country, where birds perched on a branch speak, their songs echo through the valleys, carried along by fresh breezes.

We can marvel at waves foaming soon after they break close to shore while allowing fine white sand to tickle our toes, internalizing how this feels – and slow down and take it all in. Every action we take, thought we have, decision we make can have a profound effect on ourselves and the world around us.

Does this disease give us an opportunity to care for each other with compassion? Yes, it does. We have learned how to ease suffering, extend life, provide hope and so much more. Generosity abounds from so many people freely giving money to causes, but can we find what we all want? A cure for this relentless disease.

2 7

APPROACHING WHERE I STAND NOW

The "well patient journey" Dr. Linda Reynolds aspires to is different than other forms of alternative medicine. This approach views all our systems: emotional body, energy body, physical body, spiritual body and miasmatic (genetic predisposition) and the interaction and synergy between them.

The process begins by reading the DNA in one's blood. Priorities are established, treatment plans are in place and the journey to synchronize all systems is introduced. Detoxification is a major ongoing process and critical to remove what the body may work so hard to eliminate, thus restoring its energy, encouraging rebalancing. Another focus is attempting to change one's environment.

My expectation as I grow older, to remain in a state of good health relevant to my age, is reasonable. My travels have taken me here and I have faith that this is exactly where I'm supposed to be right now.

Western medicine aims to combat disease by using drugs or surgery. It definitely has a place in our society. In emergencies, well-trained physicians can work wonders. Technological advances clearly show disease, broken bones can be set to heal, surgeries can give new life by replacing aging, fragile hips, other body parts, even organs. All in an effort to alleviate pain and extend life.

In my mid 30s, a family dentist suggested removing four impacted wisdom teeth. He believed it was prudent to eliminate the possibility of future infection. When he told me there's a 20 percent chance of permanent nerve damage and numbing around my lips, I declined.

In my early 40s, during my peak running years, a torn meniscus prevented me from walking without pain. As reluctant as I was to have surgery, the only way to continue running was to do so. The recovery was as advertised. Four weeks of rehab, back on the road and in good form.

Similar results 16 years later. An innocent cough produced a bulge inches away from my midsection, signaling a hernia in need of repair. Of course, my initial reluctance to surgery accompanied time researching alternatives. Desiring to remain active, I felt my best option was surgery. No time in the gym for six weeks or so, walking led to hiking, back to working out a few months later.

Western medicine restored my ability to be as active as I had been, for the most part, without compromising my lifestyle for long periods of time. Yet, I have decided to adapt to the limitations and occasional pain stemming from a dislocated shoulder suffered in my youth. While I elected to have arthroscopic knee and hernia surgery, I have also chosen to make modifications while learning to live without surgery and six months to a year rehabilitating my shoulder.

These were not life or death choices. Even so, I considered them all very carefully. I understand that we may not have options when faced with a cancer diagnosis, or so it can appear, and electing to do nothing can be a death sentence. I imagine some conclude this is best for them. I respect you. Who knows what circumstances lead to this conclusion? Depression, discovering you have cancer late in life, even intuition. Hopefully you're finding and listening to your inner voice and learning to speak up for yourself, especially in the face of contrasting opinions.

Some may choose chemotherapy or radiation. Others may choose surgery. I honor your choices. Your journey may mirror mine, but when dreams appear or thoughts and feelings emerge, we are alone finding our own way, as we consider the uncertainty of our futures.

We can embrace the support of our children, parents, extended families and friends. We can seek advice and knowledge, decide for ourselves what is real, what to believe and whom to trust. We can avail ourselves of the multitude of organizations, groups, societies and foundations that have been created with the best intentions, over so many years, as this disease refuses to retreat, subside. Vanish.

LOOKING EVERYWHERE BUT RIGHT HERE

Our life's journey begins to materialize when we recognize that we are on it. Personal growth within the work we do for ourselves can be the impetus for global change.

My work required moving within, finding myself in quiet moments; reflecting, making connections, attempting to understand until I exhausted my resources. I can then breathe and listen to a single thought, belief, or the universe letting me know that all I do will lead me to and give me the strength to be secure in my convictions. I will then know the truth on a deeper level as the answers begin to appear.

How do I strike those aspects of my early childhood tapes from the record, allow for reprogramming or can I simply live in my conscious mind and in every moment? I continue to learn and remain open to practicing what I have found: meditation, yoga, mindfulness – and what I have yet to discover. Embracing more ways to give back, perhaps volunteering for a cause I'm passionate about, continuing to write, maybe even Buddhism. Who knows?

For now, I find myself viewing how I spend my time and other resources, dedicating this part of my health journey to what I have discovered two years ago when visiting Dr. Linda Reynolds. I believe this is far better than submitting to harmful therapies and toxic chemicals. These compromising, often drawn out traditional therapies come with short-term and potentially irreversible, long-term side effects.

I am so tuned into this sensitive body and have much information from my years of researching as well as an active, sometimes neurotic imagination. Therefore, it can be difficult to completely ignore a new pain (probably due to age) or a potential symptom of prostate cancer. For now, I am working toward full acceptance that the best way to eliminate worry and anxiety is to forgo extending my arm and making a fist. It has been two and a half years. No appointments with Dr. Martin or Dr. Sperling. No more research. I know this may not sound prudent, but I'm convinced that if I did bloodwork, and found a rising PSA, I would not consider conventional treatment.

And yet, as I go deeper, it's possible that just like my mom said, "I don't want to go yet," if I'm facing health challenges as I age or sense that my time is near, I might not be so resolute in my convictions. I may so dearly value life that compromises to the quality of it would be welcomed.

We do not have the control we would like to think we have. Much as I didn't when I discovered my dad's shadow touched mine. I can spend time foraging through data, take what I learn, modify it as needed, and hope the desired goals come to fruition. Knowing I have done my part, I can then let go of the outcome. The end of the journey gives us a moment to breathe and reflect as we move to the next adventure. But, it's the lessons along the way, and what we do with them, that feed our soul. It really *is* about the journey. So, if much of this is about dying, or the fear of dying, then I want to let go of that. I already know the ending. Watchful waiting does not have to be an option.

I am guided by intuition. I am committed to remembering what I am thankful for – the body I elected to inhabit, the lessons I came here to complete and free will – the vehicle of my choices. Every day is a gift. I am grateful for all my earthly experiences and for whatever exists beyond that.

Perhaps finding myself may have been as simple as looking in that mirror 53 years ago, my father beside me, his arm resting on my shoulder. If it meant looking into my hazel eyes until I saw my soul, knowing forgiveness and gratitude would lead me down a different path, would my life have been so different? I imagine so. But whatever lessons would have materialized, difficult decisions made, heartaches, joy, love and loss finding their way, I believe my approach would have been similar.

I'm still finding myself, but I have a much better sense of what that is. A peace-loving soul with strong values and beliefs. A seeker. A man struggling to keep his heart open, discovering how to do so with compassion and kindness. Intolerant of injustice, inequality and learning how to speak my truth softly yet convincingly. Stepping outside myself to help others. Hopefully, taking pen to paper is a beginning. Patience, believing that surrendering to the universal flow is far better than accelerating onto the highway of life, anticipating every turn, worrying if I will find a way to my desired outcome.

To have the awareness to know who I am, that I will challenge you with my words, attempting to convince anyone that violence, hatred and war are not credible alternatives. To have the wisdom to know when my message falls on deaf ears and turn away. To recognize that when large-scale change seems to be taking forever, I just don't have the patience and can lose faith.

I believe there are no coincidences. Every action I have taken, each person I have met, all my experiences have brought me to where I am right now. Everything I have done has led me back to myself.

Have I been looking everywhere but right here?

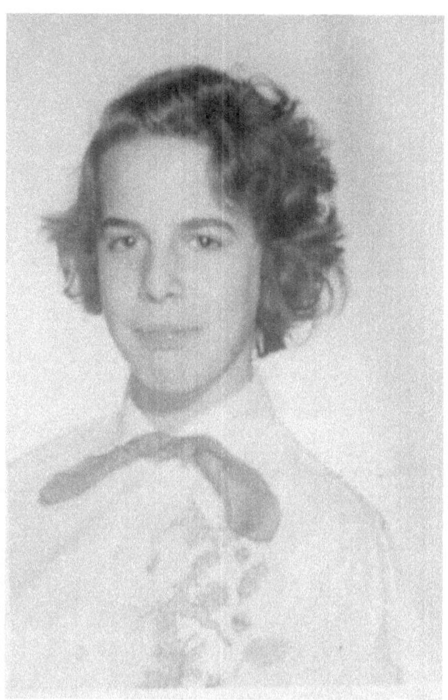

Fifty four years, I was on the receiving end of my sister's long standing, uncomplicated love and affection.

This book is dedicated in memory of Ronda Kalish, who lived this way and by example served others.

RESOURCES

I have learned much over the years from researching prostate cancer, talking with Dr. Thomas Martin, Dr. Dan Sperling, other physicians, and friends. The following resources provided me with valuable information.

Websites:

Cancer Tutor – www.cancertutor.com – a resource tool that includes information about alternative doctors, preventive approaches as well as unconventional treatments.

National Cancer Institute – www.cancer.gov — Up-to-date cancer information from the U.S. government's agency for cancer research.

Web MD – www.webmd.com – Publisher of news and information pertaining to human health.

Prostate Cancer Foundation – www.pcf.org – Provides research to improve the prevention, detection and treatment of prostate cancer.

Cancer *Care* – www.cancercare.org – Provides support for people with cancer, caregivers, loved ones and the bereaved.

Prostate Cancer Research Institute – www.pcri.org – Helps men and caregivers research prostate cancer treatment options.

Us TOO – www.ustoo.org – A site for wives, partners and family members providing information, counseling and educational meetings with the goal of assisting men with prostate cancer.

Man to Man – www.ncb.nlm.nih.gov – A source for support groups for men with prostate cancer.

Women Against Prostate Cancer – www.menshealthnetwork.org – An advocacy organization supporting women and their families

Some tests for prostate cancer:

The Gleason Score, based on tissue samples obtained from a biopsy, is the information used to determine the stage and aggressiveness of prostate cancer. The lower the score, the closer the sample is to normal prostate tissue and the tumor is less likely to spread. A higher score increases the probability the cancer will spread. The first number assigned is the grade that is most common in the tumor. The most promising Gleason score is 3+3=6 indicating a lower grade early-stage, nonaggressive cancer. Next is 3+4=7. This typically has a good outlook where 4+3 is more likely to grow and spread but less likely to do so than a score of 8. Gleason scores of 9 or 10 have the worst outlook. Source: Medical News Today

A Prostate Specific Antigen (PSA) test, measures two different forms of PSA; free and bound or total. The general opinion is the higher amount of free PSA the lower the chance for cancer. Source: Cancer Research-UK.

MRI guided biopsy targets select tissue revealed by the MRI imaging. Typically, fewer samples are needed than a biopsy without an MRI, and the images appear in finer detail. Source: Sperling Prostate Center.

PET scans produce multidimensional images using a dye that can be swallowed or injected into a vein that can reveal the presence and stage of cancer, showing whether and where it has spread and help determine treatment. PET scans come with the risk of radiation exposure. Source: Medical News Today.

C-reactive protein blood test measures a nonspecific marker for inflammation. Source: Purely Living.

PCA3 Urine Test can determine if elevated PSA levels are likely caused by prostate cancer. Source: Healthline.

Treatment Options

Brachytherapy or seed implantation works internally when radioactive material is placed inside the prostate. Source: www.mayoclinic.org

External beam radiation uses high energy beams such as x-rays and protons to kill cancer cells. These treatments include *Intensified-Modulated radiation therapy (*IMRT*) and three-dimensional conformal radiation therapy* (3-D conformal RT). Source: www.mayoclinic.org

Proton therapy uses a focused ray of proton particles to destroy cancerous tissues. The treatment is capable of delivering high doses of radiation to accurately target cancer cells. Source: Loma Linda University.

SBRT (CyberKnife) a form of external beam radiation delivering high doses of radiation with extreme accuracy. Source: www.Healthline.com

Some treatments use different sources of energy to attack cancer cells:

High Intensity Focused Ultrasound (HIFU) uses soundwaves to create heat as a specific point, the heat destroying the target tissue. HIFU research began in the 1950s. Source: HIFU prostate services

Cryosurgery or cryoablation a procedure recommended for men who have been previously treated for prostate cancer when the cancer returns. It uses extreme cold to freeze the prostate, so the cancer cells within it will die. Source: www.my.clevelandclinic.org

Hormone therapy or androgen suppression therapy can reduce levels of male hormones in the body and stop them from affecting prostate cancer cells. Androgens, a male sex hormone stimulate the growth of prostate cancer cells. Source: American Cancer Society

Focal Laser Ablation is a procedure using a 3T multi-parametric MRI and thermal energy to destroy the cancer. Source: Sperling Prostate Center

Vascular targeted photodynamic therapy (VTP), destroys tumors and the blood vessels that support them by delivering the intravenous drug Tookad. Source: www. prostatecancerinfolink.net

Some centers that offer alternative and traditional therapies:

Hippocrates Health Institute, West Palm Beach, Florida provides programs for healthy lifestyle changes focusing on raw vegan food, holistic therapies, psychotherapy, fitness and whole food supplementation.

The Schachte Center for Complementary Medicine, Rockland County, New York combines innovative ideas, nutrition and holistic health using alternative, integrative and complementary medical care.

An Oasis of Healing, Meza, Arizona takes an integrative, alternative approach to treating cancer.

The Skilling Institute, Phoenix, Arizona approaches alternative cancer therapy with the Photon Genie and Photon Genius Super Sauna.

If my journey touches you, please feel free to reach out to me at leskalish@hotmail.com

ACKNOWLEDGMENTS

To my sons, Bryan and Evan, you both changed my life forever when you came into this world. For that I am eternally grateful. I love you.

To Mary, knowing you're always there has taught me more than you know and has given me the freedom to follow my heart. I love you.

To Susan, your desire to type my chicken scratch leaves me wanting to write more. To our friendship.

Thank you to my first readers Liz, Valerie, Linda, Phil, Amy, Mark, Jen, Rod, Randy, Nancy and Ramzey. Your thoughts, advice and suggestions were constant reminders, guiding me through this process.

To my developmental editor Nickey, the challenges you placed before me stretched my awareness, opening me to a deeper understanding.

To my copy editor, Jen W., thank you for adding a bright light to this adventure. Your expertise, thoroughness, persistence and willingness to work together has helped unfold layers, bringing my beliefs into a clearer focus. Getting to know you better has been a gift.

To K.R. Conway (Kate), the Taskmaster. A best-selling Urban Fantasy novelist, graphic designer, and book publisher, she always knew there was more to do. You guided me through the final step, taking my manuscript and transforming it into a book I am proud to share.

We would rather be playing in the streets of Bensonhurst than dressing up for our 5th grade graduation. On the front, let me introduce you to my best friend, Little Tim. To my left is Robert Finkelstein. The least goofy boy in the middle, is me. On the back jacket are my parents, Max and Edith, standing in front of our mammoth 1956 Chevy, circa 1958 Brooklyn, New York.

ABOUT THE AUTHOR

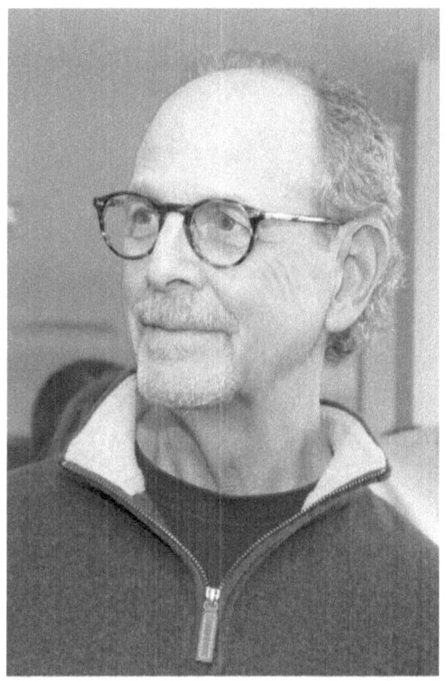

Les, his wife Mary and their golden retriever, Charley, live on Cape Cod. The beauty that surrounds them is enhanced by Les's passion for landscaping and gardening. When the winds howl and the temperatures fall, the warmth of Fort Myers Beach calls. Both places lure family and friends year-round.